African Hairstyles

Styles of Yesterday and Today

Esi Sagay

HEINEMANN
LONDON IBADAN NAIROBI

Heinemann Educational Books Ltd
22 Bedford Square, London WC1B 3HH
PMB 5205, Ibadan · PO Box 45314, Nairobi
PO Box 61581, Marshalltown 2107, RSA

EDINBURGH MELBOURNE AUCKLAND
HONG KONG SINGAPORE KUALA LUMPUR
NEW DELHI KINGSTON PORT OF SPAIN

Heinemann Educational Books Inc.
4 Front Street, Exeter,
New Hampshire 03833, USA

British Library Cataloguing in Publication Data
Sagay, Esi
    African hairstyles: styles of yesterday and today.
    1. Hairdressing – Africa – History
    I. Title
    646.7'242'096   TT958

ISBN 0 435 89830 2

The Book Society of Canada Ltd.,
4386 Sheppard Avenue East,
Agincourt, Ontario MIS 3B6.

ISBN 0 7725 0011 8

Designed by Christie Archer

Typeset in 11/12pt Souvenir by Crawley Composition Ltd, Crawley, Sussex
Printed in Great Britain by BAS Printers Ltd, Over Wallop, Hampshire

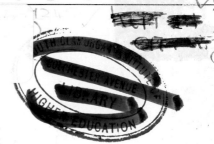
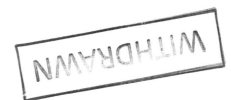

This book is dedicated
to all those whose love,
kindness and encouragement
have been a source
of constant inspiration.

My Parents
Gabriel Amone Sagay
Comfort Buwa Sagay

and the following

Chief and Mrs Ayo Rosiji
Dr Abimbola Silva
Omodele Karunwi
Andrew A E Sagay

Contents

Acknowledgements   ix

Introduction   xi

Styles of Yesterday   1
Ancient Egypt   3
North Africa   5
West Africa – the Sahel   9
Tropical West Africa   19
Central Africa   23
East Africa   29
Southern Africa   35
Malagasy Republic   41

Styles of Today   45
Cornrowing   49
How to cornrow   51
Cornrowing with an attachment   60
Men's styles   63

Hair Threading   65
The design parted on the scalp   66
The design on threaded strands   68
How to thread hair   72
Caucasian & Oriental hairstyles   88

Combined Cornrowing   90
& Hair Threading

Haircare   105

Bibliography   108

Acknowledgements

This book has been in preparation for seven years and during this time many debts have been incurred which I should like to acknowledge. These range from close friends and relatives to casual acquaintances and various other contributors.

Firstly, I should like to thank Dr Joe Okpaku for his encouragement and guidance during the early stages of the book; also Grace Feliciano and Bennie Arrington.

My special thanks to Salimatu Diallo of the Organization of African Unity office in New York; Lena Gueye of the Senegalese National Assembly; Babatunde Olatunji of the Centre for African Culture, Haarlem, New York; Black Civil Rights activist Stockely Carmichael; Tina Phillips of New York; the late South African Nationalist David Sebeko – for their keen interest and assistance.

For their help and useful advice, educationist Phebian Ogundipe, Dr Ekpo Eyo, Director of Museums and Monuments in Nigeria, Mr Arinze and Mrs V Ugbodaga of the Lagos museum.

I am grateful to the following for their contributions in numerous ways: Bose Clarke, Dan Agbakoba, Dapo Odebiyi, Gbite Olagbegi-Wilcox, Saint John Jesse Nuno, Flora Odebiyi, Susie Chin, Rita Hogan, Agnes Amarvi, Molara Marquis-Mims and Josephine Apiafi.

My thanks to Karen Nangle of Photo Researchers, Sally Jane Gluckson of Freelance Photographers Guild and Ken Burger of Black Star, all of New York, and to the following institutions: Library of Congress, Washington DC; Brooklyn Library, New York; The Museum of Natural History; New York Public Library; Columbia University Library, New York; Bettman Archive; National Museum, Benin City; Federal Ministry of Social Development, Youth, Sports and Culture.

Immense thanks to Emil Keffa of the Ivory Coast Ministry of Foreign Affairs for the translations of research material from French and German into English, Betty Webb for very kindly typing the manuscript, Irene Woolridge, Sharon Crawford, Debra, Nadel and Iya Ozuka for cornrowing some of the styles.

My sincere thanks to James Currey of HEB London and all other members of staff who have worked on this book. To Aig Higo, Akin Thomas, Mrs Akanni and all other members of the HEB Ibadan, Nigeria for all their kindness and help.

Most of all, I am greatly indebted to all the wonderful models and photographers, whose patience and co-operation have made it possible for this book to materialise.

The author and publisher would like to thank the following for permission to reproduce photographs in this book:

American Museum of Natural History, New York for no. 24; Alex Amagatcher for nos. 109, 112 and 127; Caroline Amato for no. 150; Bennie Arrington for drawing nos. 3, 4 and 7; Babs Photo Stars, Ibadan for no. 51; Bassey for nos. 95, 99a-e, 100a-e and 149a-b; Black Star, New York for nos. 12, 25, 26, 40, 43 and 46; Stockley Carmichael for no. 19; Director of Information, S.A. Consulate General for nos. 39, 41, 42, 44 and 45; Federal Ministry of Social Development, Youth, Sports and Culture, Lagos for nos. 14 and 21; Norman Fredrick for nos. 60a-b, 61a-b, 62, 63, 64, 65, 66a-c, 67, 68, 69a-b, 70, 71, 72a-c, 73, 74a-b, 75a-d, 81, 82, 83a-b, 85, 86, 87, 88, 89, 92, 93, 94, 98a-g, 101a-b, 102a-b, 104a-b, 105a-b, 106, 107, 108a-b, 110a-b, 111, 113, 114, 115a-b, 116a-b, 117a-b, 118, 119a-b, 122, 123, 124, 125, 126, 128a-b, 129, 130a-b, 132a-b, 133a-b, 134, 135, 136, 139, 140a-b, 141, 142, 143, 144a-b, 145, 146a-b and 147; Freelance Photographers Guild, Inc., New York for nos. 22, 32, 48, 49 and 50; Dave Greene for nos. 120a-b; The John Hillelson Agency Ltd., for nos. 27 and 28; Ibanga's (Never-Rest) Studio, Lagos, for nos. 55 and 59; Sarah Nuno for no. 91; Christo Odion for nos. 90, 96, 97, 103a-c and 131a-b; Nancy Palmer Photo Agency for no. 17; Photo Researchers, Inc., New York for nos. 2, 5, 6, 8, 9, 10, 11, 13, 15, 16, 18, 23, 29, 30, 31, 33, 34, 35, 36, 37 and 38; Bayo Sonekan for nos. 77a-b, 78, 79, 80, 121a-b, 137a-b, 138 and 148a-b.

Introduction

African hair sculpture is an art. Africans rarely leave the hair or the body in their simple, natural state but spend a considerable amount of time and energy on grooming and self-adornment. The hair has always been accorded particular attention.

The art of hairdressing in Africa is practised almost exclusively by women, although male hairdressers can be found in some areas. This domestic skill, which has been handed down from generation to generation, requires artistry, manual dexterity and patience, as many styles are elaborate and time-consuming. For the traditional hairdresser, hair is a medium for creative self-expression.

Hair is styled for a number of reasons: in some parts of the African continent different styles distinguish age sets; in others ceremonial occasions are marked by special styles; often, as is the case elsewhere in the world, fashion dictates the ways in which the hair is worn. The design and construction of hair sculpture call on techniques as varied as the styles themselves. Some coiffures depend on the use of sisal or clay, the bark of trees or cloth pads; others involve the intricate knitting, braiding and threading of the hair. The most complex styles, which may take the hairdresser anything from several hours to whole days to complete, are now found only in the interior of the continent (in the so-called 'primitive' parts of Africa), where people still live in a manner that grants them the leisure to practise the art of elaborate hair sculpture; in urban areas traditional hairdressers who employ the less demanding techniques of hair braiding and threading can be found side by side with those who have adopted Western styles.

In a discussion of the hairstyles of Africa it is helpful to divide the continent into two parts by an imaginary line running from Dakar, Senegal, in the west to Khartoum, Sudan, in the east. To the north of this line live the light-skinned, straight-haired Hamites and Semites of North Africa. Around the dividing line, which covers the Sahelian region of Africa, the inhabitants tend to have brown skins and curly hair as a result of Semite– or Hamite–Negroid intermixtures. South of the line live the dark-skinned, kinky-haired members of the black race. Given the fact that Africa is a vast continent, inhabited by peoples of divergent backgrounds who differ physically, linguistically and culturally, nothing that is said or written about any part can be true of the whole. Each region has its own traditional styles; each group of people has its own code of aesthetics, which distinguishes it among the multitude of ethnic groups.

In the first part of this book, in order to provide a bird's-eye view, the traditional hairstyles of Africa are categorized in very broad terms. After a discussion of hair fashion in ancient Egypt, styles are grouped by region to represent those of the North, the Sahel, the tropical West, Central, East and Southern Africa and the Malagasy Republic (formerly Madagascar). The second part of the book deals with hairstyles of today, particularly the popular techniques of cornrowing and hair threading.

Styles of
Yesterday

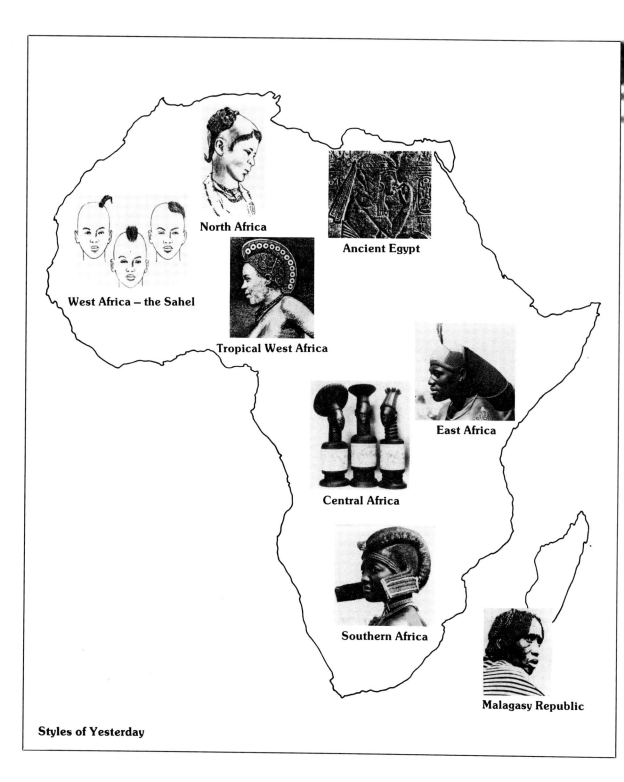

North Africa

Ancient Egypt

West Africa — the Sahel

Tropical West Africa

East Africa

Central Africa

Southern Africa

Malagasy Republic

Styles of Yesterday

Ancient Egypt

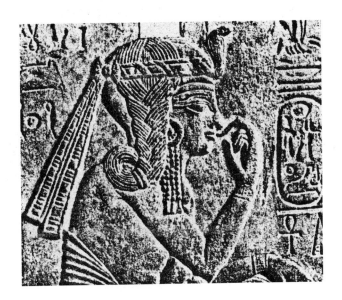

In ancient Egypt, where the conservative religious outlook of the people affected every facet of life, a very rigid code of personal appearance persisted for several centuries. Dress and hairstyle indicated social position. In the early period of this great civilization hairstyles were simple and natural, but later the customs of head shaving and wig wearing became accepted practice for men and women alike.

Priests and high-ranking officials frequently had their entire bodies shaved. Young boys were required to shave their heads except for a long, curled lock of hair over the right temple, known as the 'lock of youth'. Although this was rarely seen on girls, young princesses sometimes wore braided 'locks of youth'.

The fashion of wearing wigs, at first reserved as a status symbol for the elite, is believed to have originated in Egypt as long ago as 3000 BC. Wigs were generally constructed from human hair, wool, cotton or palm-leaf fibres and rested upon well ventilated caps. They were dyed black for everyday wear, but other dyes – green, red and blue – were used on wigs for ceremonial occasions. After a wig had been curled, twisted or braided it was usually stiffened with beeswax, which preserved the style.

Beards were generally worn without adornment; the longer the beard, the higher the status of its wearer. However, false beards fabricated in gold and braided beards were worn by the god-kings, and Egyptian queens – perhaps vying for equality with their male counterparts – also wore false beards.

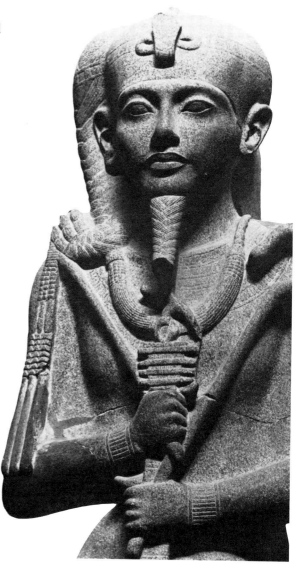

1 *previous page*
Egyptian princess wearing a braided 'lock of youth' and a circlet of the sacred serpent goddess of Lower Egypt.

2 *above*
Statue of the God Khons from the Khons Temple at Karnak, Egypt, 18th Dynasty, 1350 BC.

North Africa

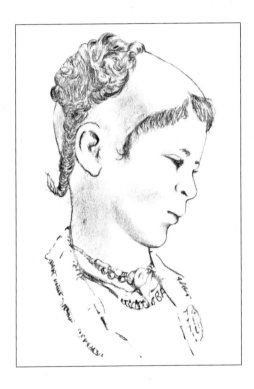

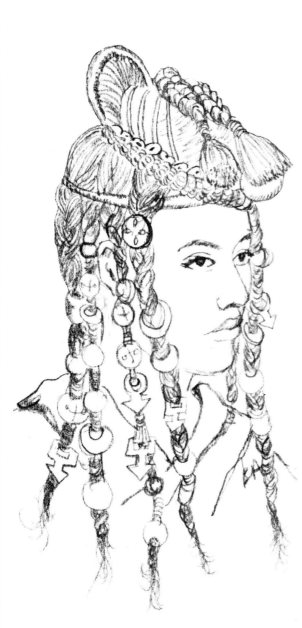

In the Mahgreb, inhabited by Tunisians, Algerians and Moroccans, men, women and children had their hair cut and arranged in accordance with the styles dictated by custom for age sets and with local, traditional beliefs.

A week after they were born baby boys had their hair shaved into tufts. They wore their hair in this style until they reached puberty, when their heads were shaved completely. As the change of hairstyle at puberty signified a change of age group, their parents often marked the occasion with a gift, such as a gun, a camel or a house.

While men wore their hair in two styles only, one before puberty and the other after, women adopted three styles, indicating childhood, adolescence and adulthood. Girls wore their hair partly shaved and partly braided from birth until they were twelve years old. In adolescence the hair was allowed to grow evenly all over the head and was braided simply. The styles of adult women were very complex, especially on ceremonial occasions, when the hair was decorated with shells, coins and other ornaments. (Some of the styles took between three and four hours to arrange.) These ornaments were omitted from the coiffure when a woman's husband was away from home.

3 *previous page*
Moroccan boy.

4 *left*
Moroccan woman.

5 *opposite*
Moroccan woman in traditional dress.

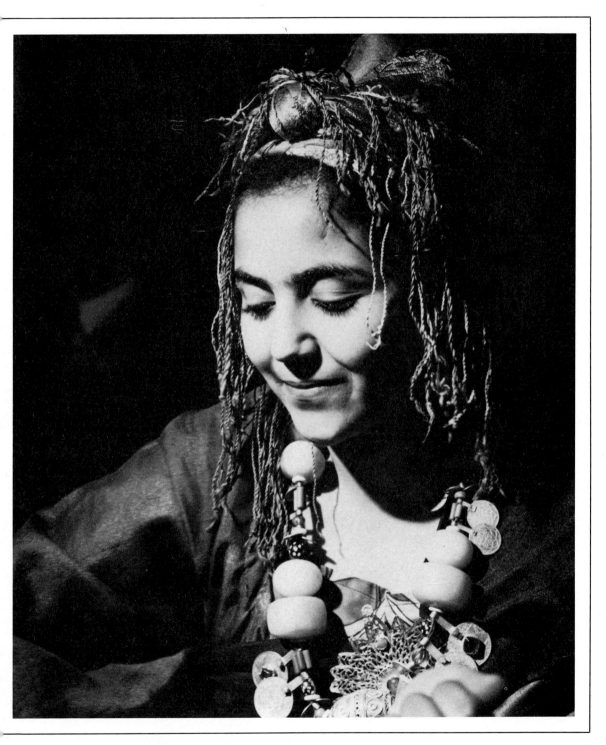

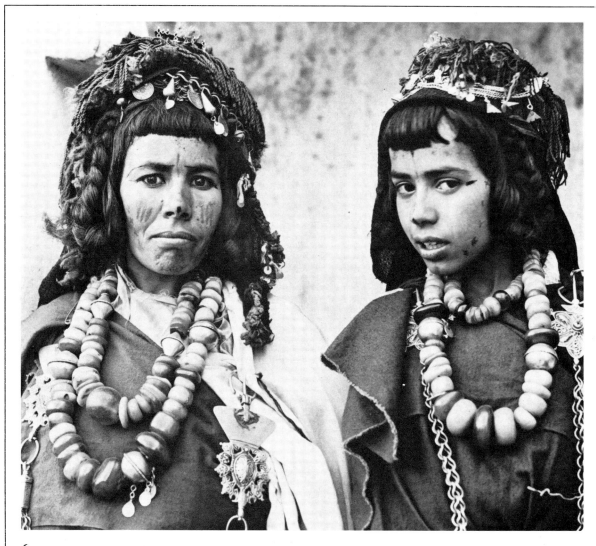

6
Berber woman and girl from the
Atlas Mountains.

West Africa
– the Sahel

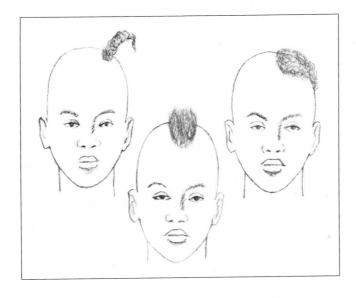

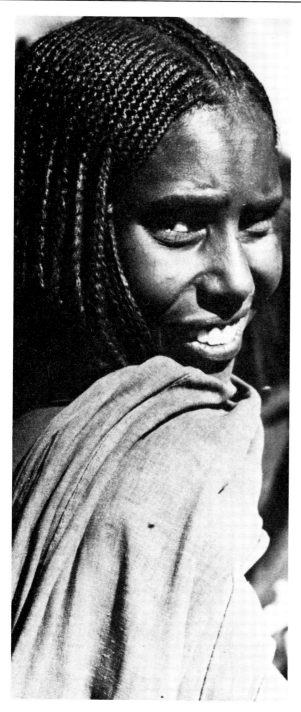

The Fulani, known as *Fulah*, *Fulbe* or *Puel*, were generally a race of Negro–Hamitic nomadic pastoralists, light brown in complexion. They occupied the semi-desert Sahelian areas of West Africa, from Mauritania, Senegal, Gambia, Guinea, Mali, Upper Volta, Niger and Chad to the Sudan, and were also to be found in the northern parts of Sierra Leone, Ghana, Togo, Dahomey, Nigeria and Cameroun. Because they were so scattered, there were considerable differences in their dress and hairstyles, which were influenced in part by their nomadic way of life, the peoples among whom they lived and the Islamic religion.

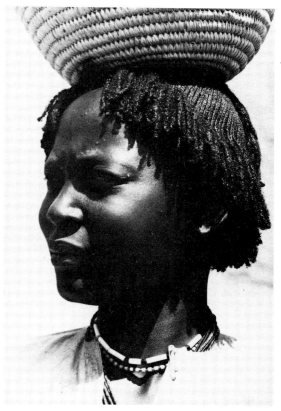

In spite of the fact that the Islamic faith required that men shave their heads and that women conceal their hair with shawls, traditional hairdressing survived. The dressing of hair began at an early age; styles were linked with clan, age set and locality. Girls had their hair cornrowed or simply braided until they married, when they wore more feminine styles. Young boys had their heads tonsured so as to leave tufts of hair in various designs, a practice that continued until they were circumcised. Having passed through this initiation into manhood, boys wore their hair in braids, which became more elaborate during the years of courtship. After marriage their heads were shaved clean.

The Fulani sometimes adopted local styles, but certain ceremonial occasions demanded very intricate traditional coiffures, which ranged from the imposing crests worn in Guinea and Mali to the exquisitely knitted hair of the Shuwa Arab women of northern Nigeria. Some of these styles were so complex and took so long to arrange that their wearers lay in the hairdresser's lap while she was working on them. Such styles were often adorned with ornaments such as cowrie shells, beads and coins.

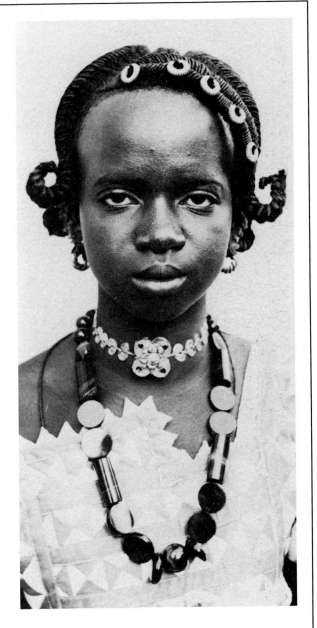

7 *page 9*
Young boys with typical Sahelian tonsures.

8 *opposite left*
Woman from the eastern region near Achebe, Chad.

9 *opposite right*
Dikwa woman from northern Cameroons.

10 *right*
Girl from Bamako, Mali.

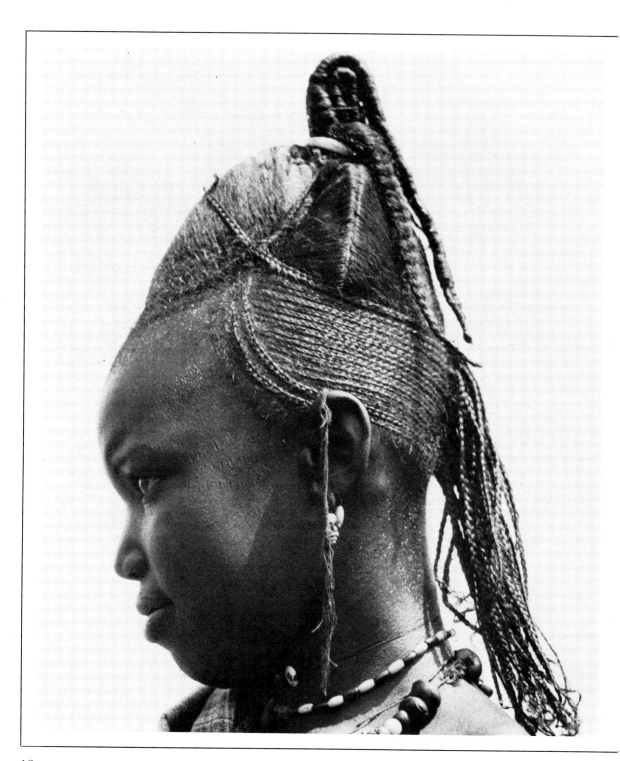

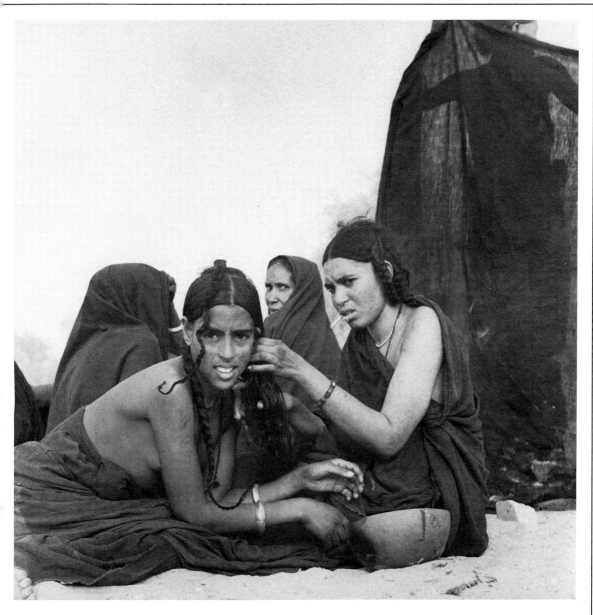

11 *opposite*
Hombori girl from Mali.

12 *above*
Hairdressing in Timbucktu, Mali.

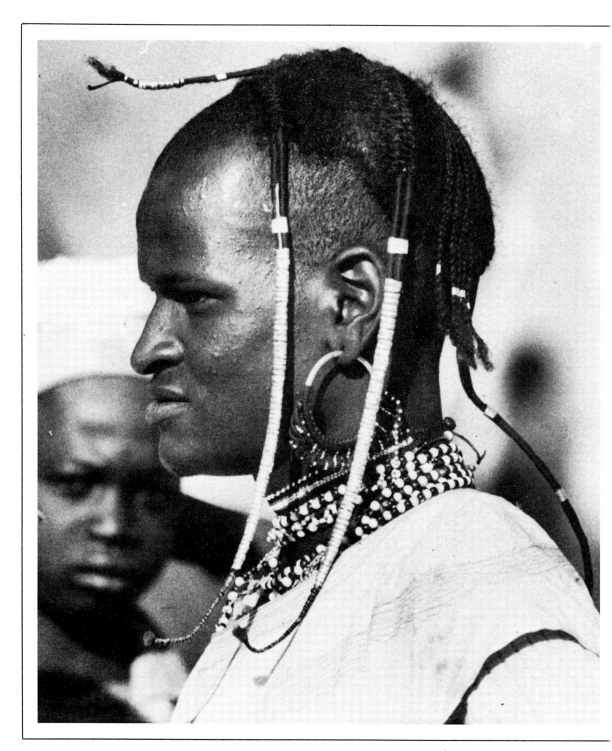

14

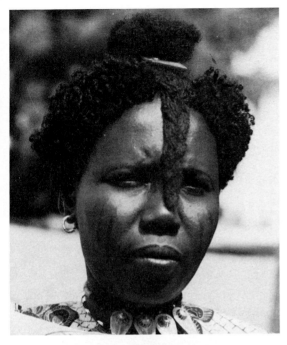

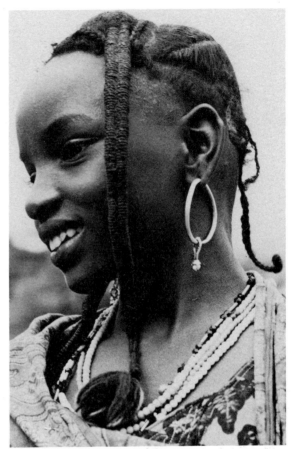

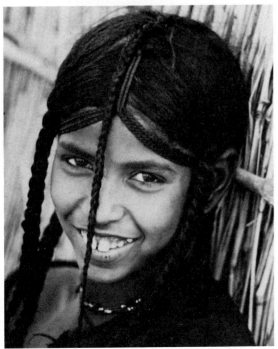

13 *opposite*
Young Fulani man from northern Nigeria. The strands of his hair are wrapped in gold.

14 *top left*
Kanuri woman from northern Nigeria.

15 *above*
Girl from Niger.

16 *bottom left*
Tuareg girl from the Azaouak Valley, Niger.

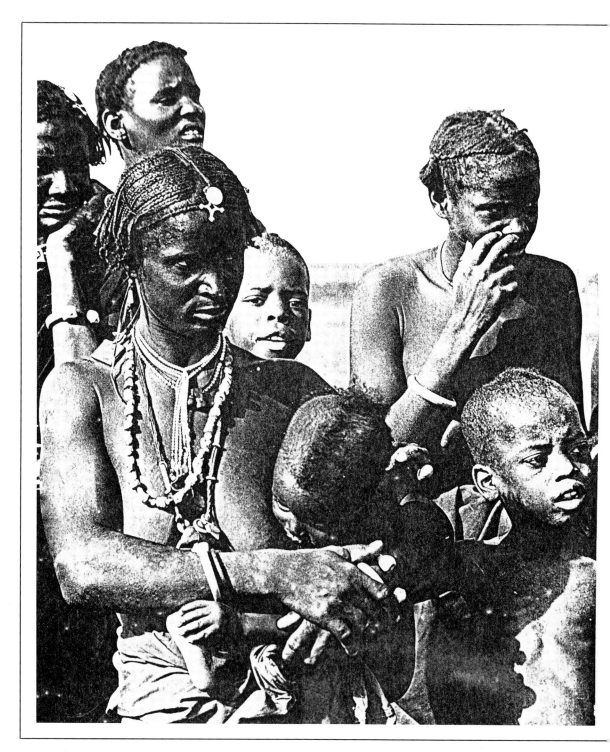

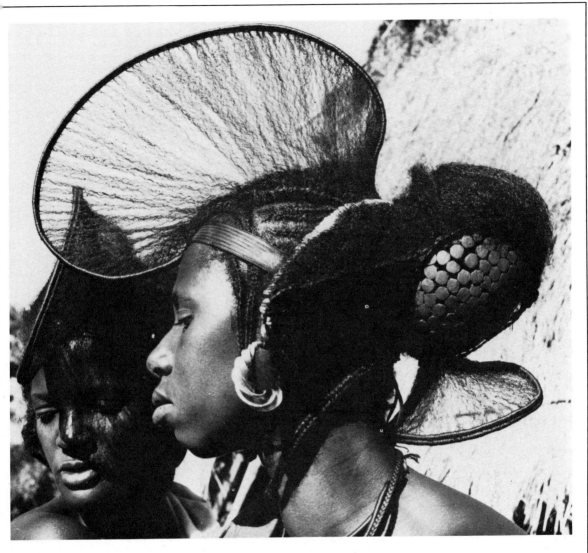

17 *opposite*
Woman from Upper Volta.

18 *above*
Fouta Djallon Peul woman from
Labe, Guinea.

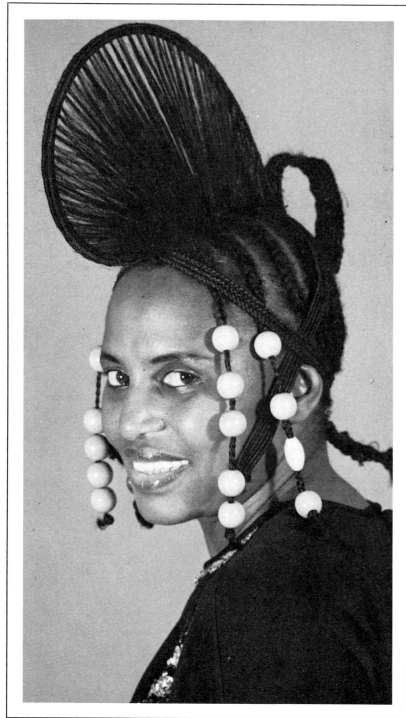

19
Miriam Makeba wearing modern interpretation of the Fouta Djallon Peul hairstyle.

Tropical
West Africa

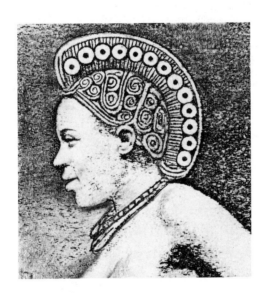

In tropical West Africa two traditional techniques for styling hair have survived to the present day – braiding (cornrowing) and hair threading, which will be discussed at greater length in the second part of this book.

Braided hair was worn in a variety of styles. The simple ones, in which women's hair was usually arranged in between four and twelve neat ridges, were worn daily; the more intricate styles were reserved for ceremonial occasions. The men generally wore their hair short, although some traditonal rulers and priests of certain religious cults braided their hair in celebration of particular festivals.

Hair threading, the more recent of the two techniques, derives its name from the process of wrapping the hair with thread. When the whole head had been threaded the hair rose from the scalp in spikes, which were sometimes left standing on end and sometimes concealed under headgear.

Among the Ibo of eastern Nigeria changing hairstyles signalled the progress of girls towards maturity. As soon as a girl's breasts began to develop she started to dress her hair with the intention of attracting the attention of men. Over a span of eight years she adopted a new style annually, each designed to display her charm and vanity. A particularly beautiful coiffure marked the day of her marriage. The hair was usually coated generously with a mixture of charcoal, clay and oil and was then moulded into a crest, which was decorated with coils of hair, coins and brass ornaments.

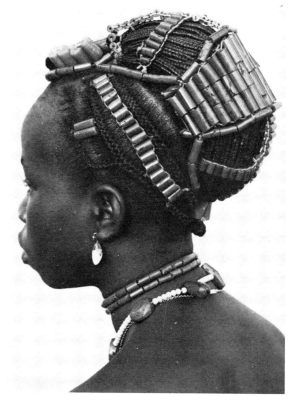

20 *previous page*
Ancient Ibo hairstyle.

21 *above*
Nigerian girl from Benin wearing the hairstyle for the Irovbode festival which is celebrated once every four years for young men and women of marriageable age.

22 *opposite*
Ibo girl from Aguleri, Nigeria. Her face, body and arms are tattooed with decorations.

23 *overleaf*
Women from Ghana.

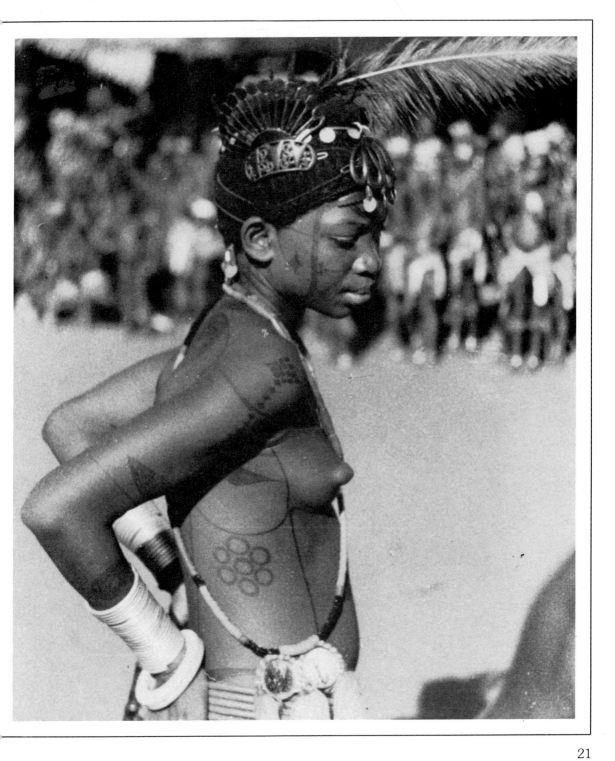

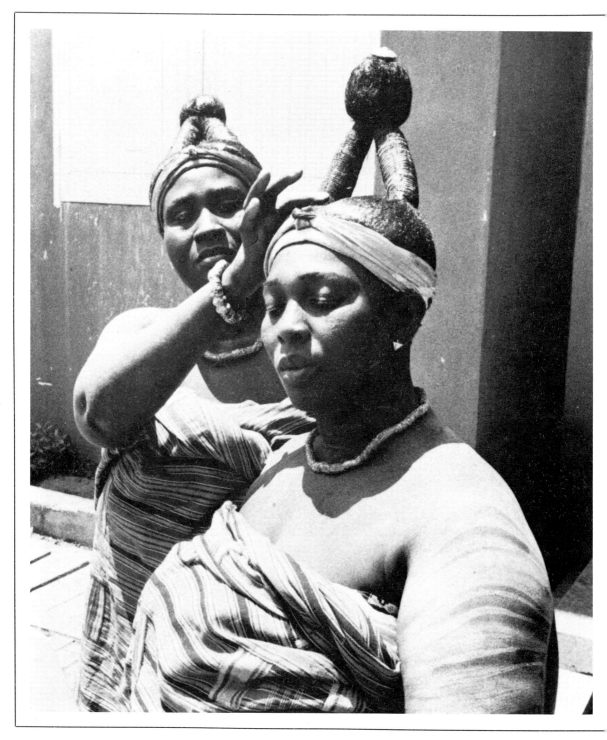

Central Africa

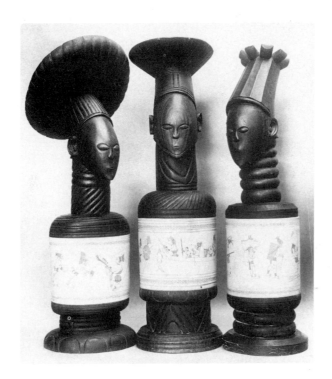

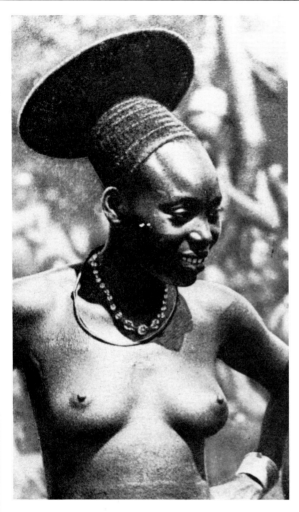

Zaïre (formerly known as the Congo) covers a large portion of Central Africa, and hair was worn in a wide variety of styles in this area.

In the Bapoto region the women were concerned primarily with styling the hair of their menfolk into cone and mitre shapes (the men usually had to lie down during this process).

Bambala women had two methods of dressing their hair: one involved shaving the front part of the head and blackening it with soot, while the hair on the back of the head was plaited into tresses and painted with a mixture of soot and palm oil; the other method was to arrange the hair in longitudinal ridges and to dye it with the aid of red ferruginous clay.

Of all the Central African styles, perhaps the most startling were those of the Mangbettu women. A unique feature of the members of this ethnic group was the shape of their heads. Mangbettu mothers pressed the heads of their babies between pieces of giraffe hide or bark, which were tied tightly around the skull. As the head grew, the head bands were replaced. The result, after years of constant wrapping and re-wrapping, was an elongated, cone-shaped cranium, which was believed to increase the brain cavity and consequently to encourage greater intelligence.

Hairstyles were devised that accentuated the shape of the head. After much of the hair had been braided and wrapped around the forehead and lower part of the head a number of times, strands of hair growing from the crown were skilfully interwoven with straw to form a cylinder, which was secured to the scalp by hairpins made out of copper, wood, ivory or bone. The fine pottery and wood carving of the Mangbettu often feature this characteristic form of hair sculpture.

24 *previous page and opposite*
Red camwood boxes featuring stylized Mangbetu hairstyles.

25 *above left*
Woman from Mangbetu, Congo.

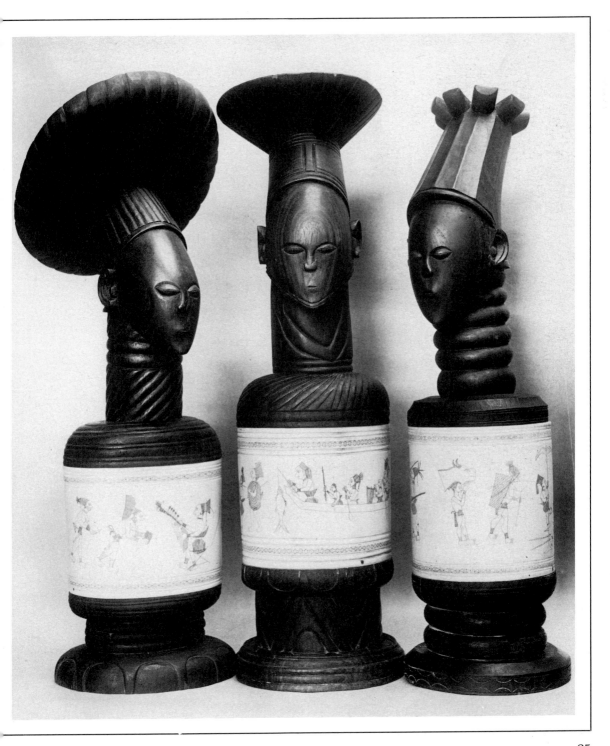

25

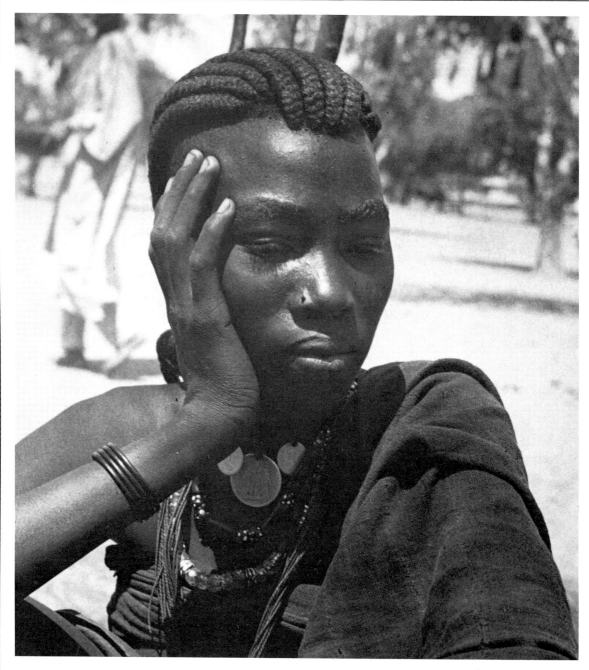

26 *above*
Sudanese woman.

27 *opposite*
Nubian girl from Messakin, Sudan.

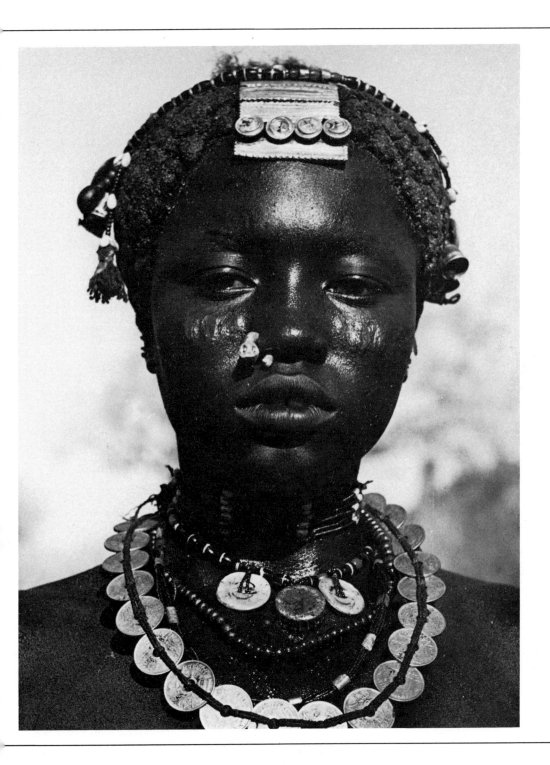

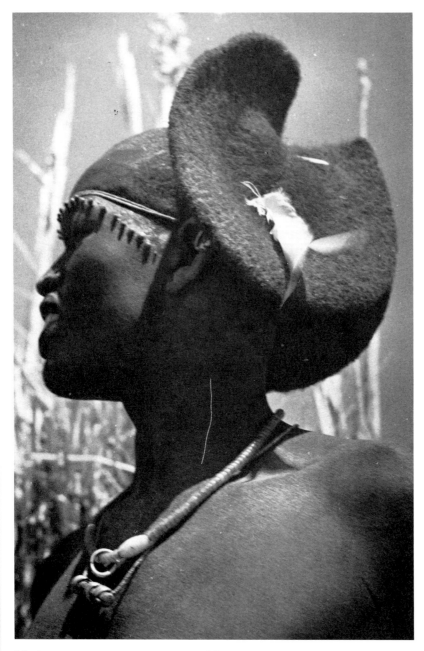

28 *above*
Shilluk herdsman from Malakal,
southern Sudan.

29 *opposite*
Karamojong man with typical
hairstyle and tattoo on his arm.

East Africa

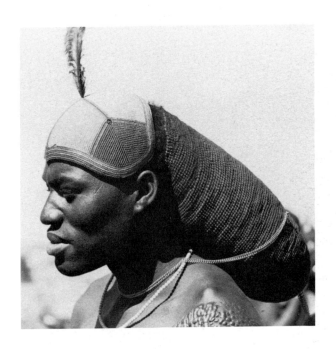

The Masai, like the Fulani of West Africa, are a nomadic people whose livelihood has always depended upon cattle. They can still be found in parts of Kenya and Tanzania.

Masai society has always placed great emphasis on personal ornament, and leisure hours were traditionally spent on grooming and self-adornment. Though local fashions varied, the styles in which hair was worn were generally much the same throughout the region.

Women usually had their heads shaved completely and smeared with a mixture of animal fat and red ochre. The typical Masai warrior, known as a *moran*, grew his hair very long and had it styled by a fellow *moran*. This arduous task sometimes took fifteen or twenty hours to perform.

First, the hair was parted from ear to ear, smeared with fat, red ochre and clay and twisted into as many as four hundred individual strands. The strands at the back of

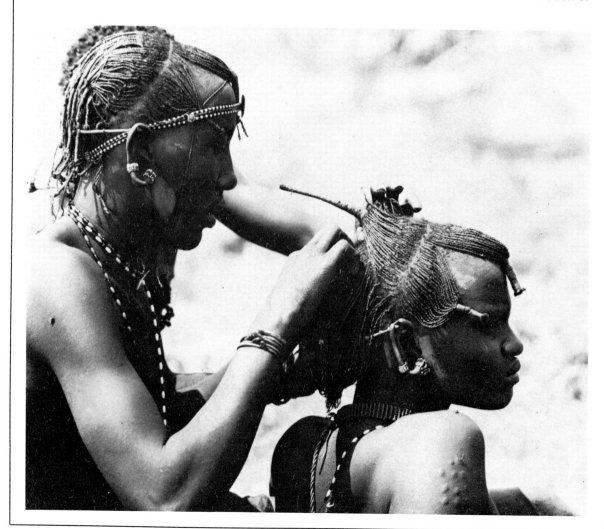

the head were then grouped into three pigtails around long, pliant sticks, and the hair ends were bound to the sticks neatly with sheep skin, so that they tapered to a point. The strands of hair at the front of the head were arranged to fall forward over the face.

30 *opposite*
Masai warrior dressing another warrior's hair.

31 *below*
Masai man and woman.

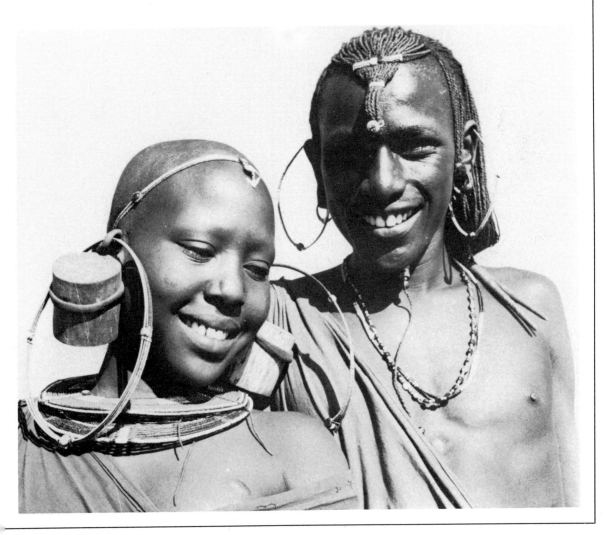

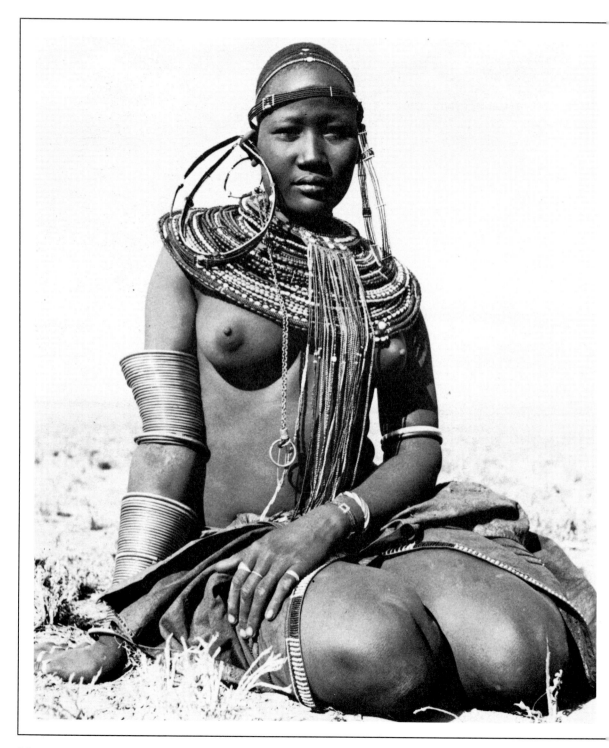

32 *opposite*
Young married Masai woman.

33 *right*
Amhara woman and child from
Allomata, Ethiopia.

34 *bottom left*
Karamojong woman from Kalapata,
Uganda.

35 *bottom right*
Nyangalom chieftain from the Omo
Valley, Ethiopia.

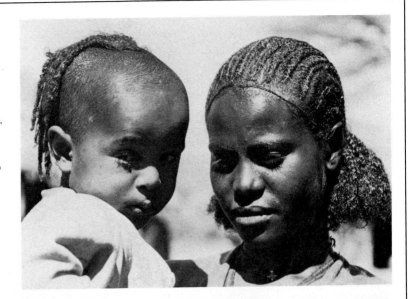

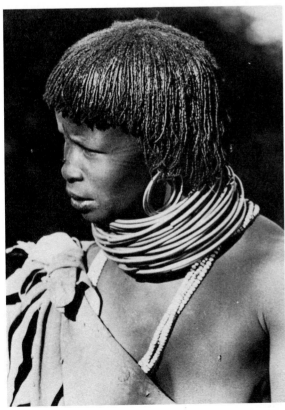

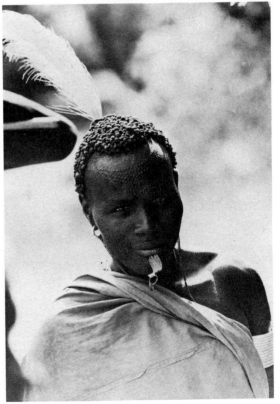

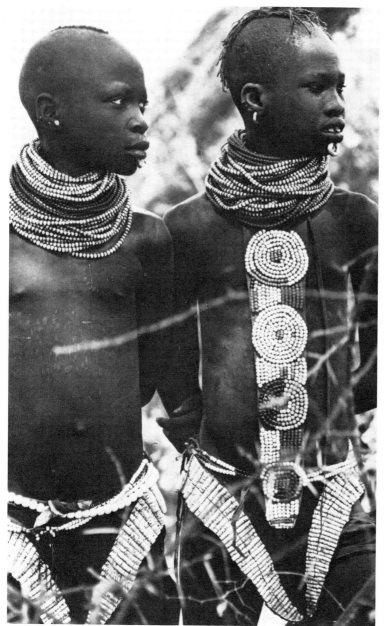

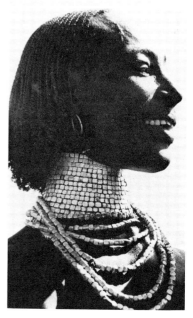

36 *left*
Nyangalom girls.

37 *above*
Borana woman from Sidamo
Province, Ethiopia.

Southern Africa

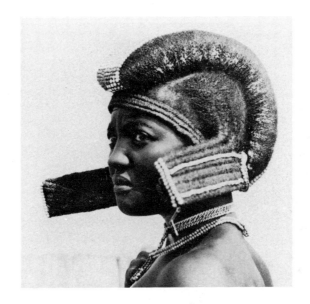

The peoples of Southern Africa adopted a very wide range of hairstyles – wider, perhaps, than that of any other part of the continent. These styles varied from tribe to tribe and even, in some cases, from village to village among the same tribe.

In Ovamboland, in the south-west, the most distinctive style was that of the marriage coiffure, which was usually made from split cow horns. It was worn like a cap and was secured to the crown of the head with clay.

The characteristic style of married women in Swaziland was the high, red-ochred topknot. The hair at the front of the head was twisted into a series of very fine curls, and the rest was tied tightly at the ends with

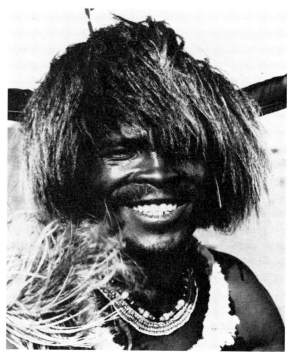

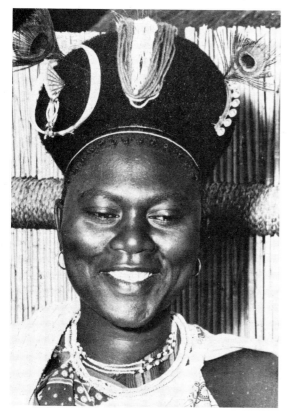

string, ochred and teased out. The central portion was then stuffed with wool or grass, very carefully rounded and stitched.

The Zulus, who lived to the south of Swaziland, were noted for their tall, ochred coiffure, which was also indicative of marital status. To create this style, red clay and fat were worked into the hair, and the entire forehead was shaved, leaving the hair on the top of the head knotted. It was often decorated with flat bones and beaded ornaments. Styles were so elaborate that head rests had to be used at times in order to preserve them intact.

39 *left*
Swazi woman with hair decorations.

38 *above*
A young man of the Swazi tribe who bleach their hair to the desired shade by applications of carbolic soap and the effect of the sun.

40
Zulu women from the Transkei.

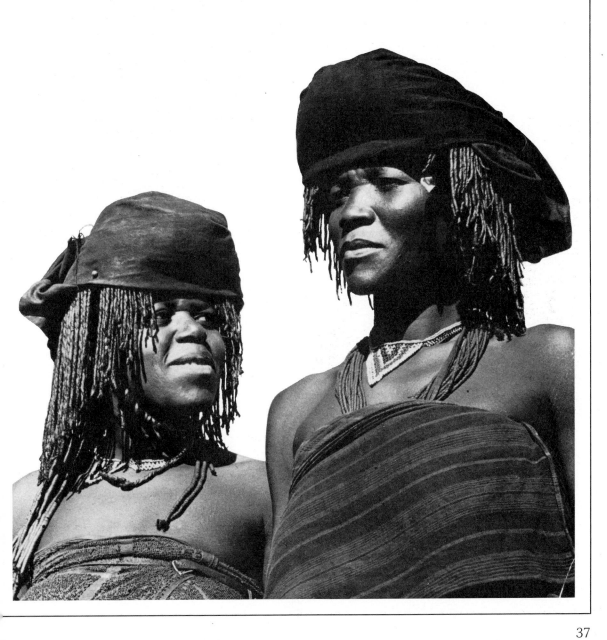

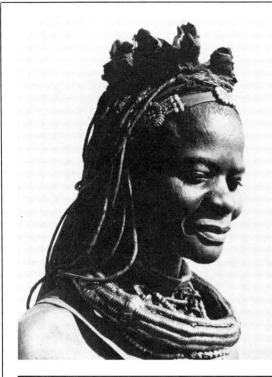

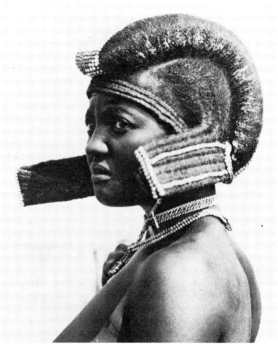

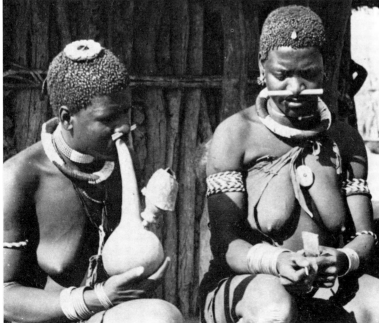

41 *top left*
Ovahimba woman, South-West Africa (Namibia).

42 *above and p. 35*
Humbi woman from the borders of Angola. The beaded hairstyle is reminiscent of an ancient Egyptian ceremonial wig or an Etruscan helmet.

43 *bottom left*
Women of the Tonga tribe, from near Choma on the Zambesi River.

44 *opposite*
Ongandjera tribeswomen of Ovambo dressing hair (Namibia).

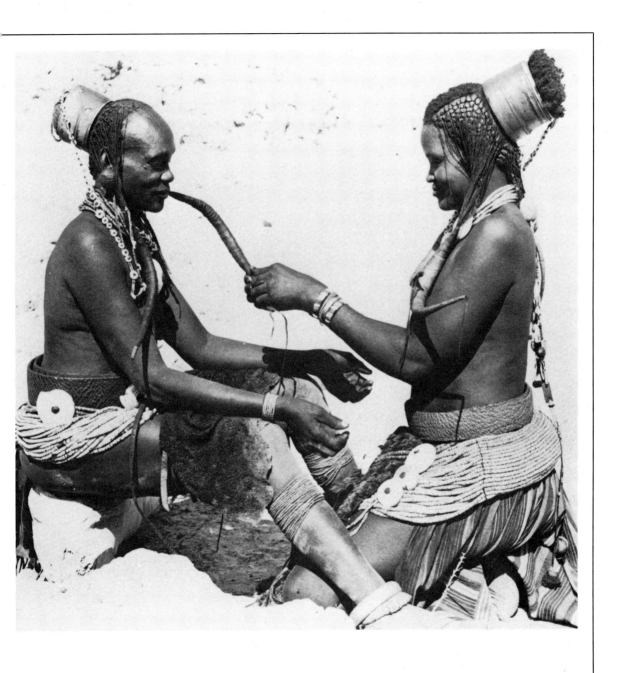

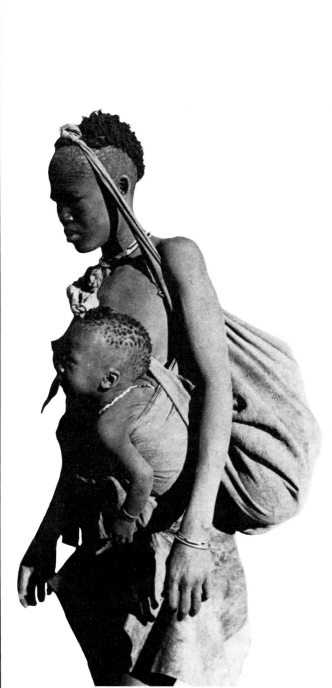

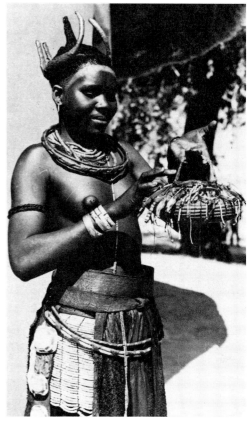

45 *above*
Ovambo woman from South-West
Africa (Namibia). She is wearing the
marriage hairstyle made from split
cow horns.

46 *left*
Woman and child of the Bushmen
tribe from the Kalahari desert,
Botswana.

47 *opposite*
Betsileo woman of the Malagasy
Republic.

Malagasy Republic

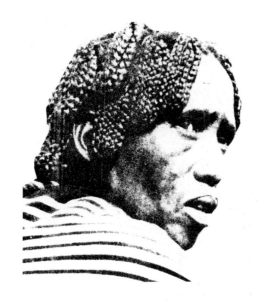

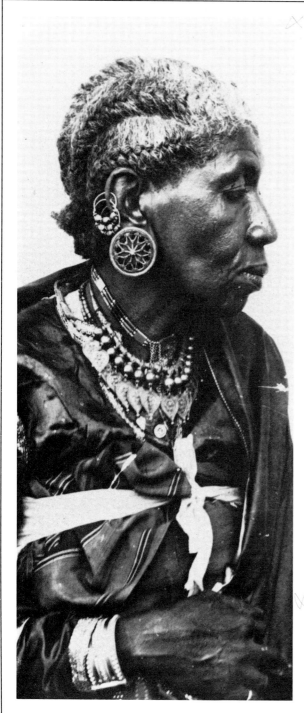

In the Malagasy Republic hairstyles varied from clan to clan, but one practice that was common to a number of ethnic groups in the central region of the island was the hair-cutting ceremony.

A child's hair remained untouched until he or she was three months old, when the parents invited guests to attend the ritual cutting of the hair. First, the hair around the child's left ear would be cut and destroyed to avert evil spirits. Then the hair around the right ear, which was believed to bring good luck, was cut, mixed with food and served to the guests. From then onwards the child's hair could be cut and shaped into any design. Boys wore their hair tonsured through adolescence and into adulthood; girls braided theirs.

Unlike the Masai of East Africa, the women of the Malagasy Republic rarely wore jewellery, which was known only in the big cities and the ports. Instead they relied on their exquisite hair styles to attract the attention of men. One of the most intricate was that of the Betsileo women, who had their hair arranged in countless single braids, designed to look like flat curls all over the head. The hair was then lavishly coated with a mixture of animal fat and honey, known as *tavo*, which gradually hardened and held the style firmly in place. If a woman was widowed, she had her head shaved in such a way that the coiffure remained intact and could later be worn as a wig.

Men also used to have their hair styled, but with the advent of French colonialism the custom was abandoned.

48 *left*
A well-to-do man of the Antalaostro tribe, Malagasy Republic.

49 *opposite*
Typical young girl from Malagasy Republic.

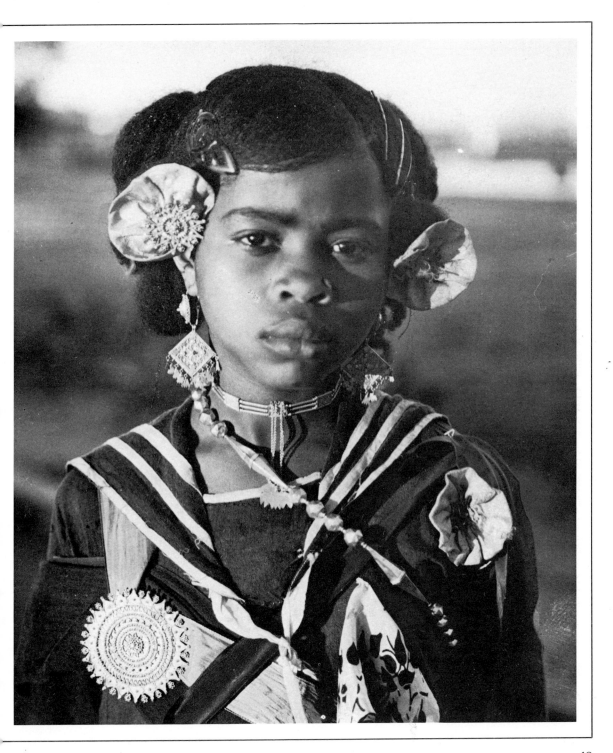

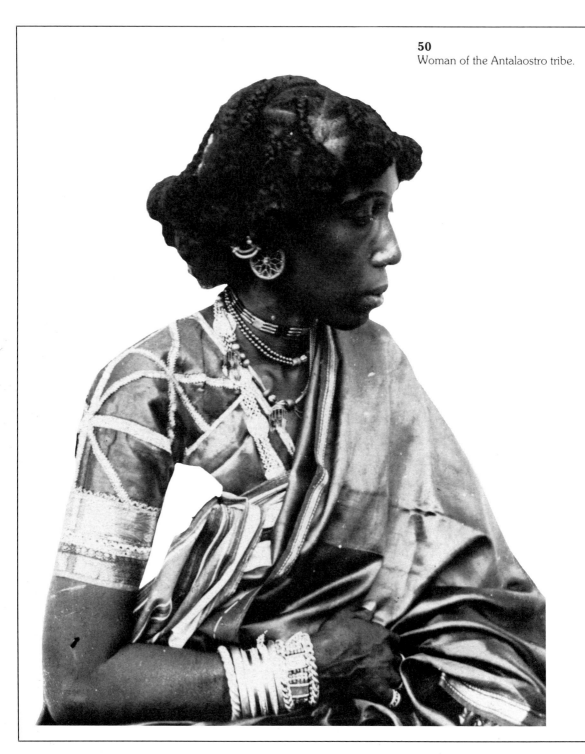

Styles of Today

Over the past fifty years Western culture has infiltrated Africa, at first in the train of the colonial administrators and educators, more recently as a consequence of the expanding empire of the mass-communication media. The changes in the domestic and social structure of many parts of the continent wrought by this external influence have been both destructive and creative.

For Africans who gradually started to see beyond the confines of the tribe, the advent of Western culture opened up avenues of contact with the outside world and stimulated fresh aspirations. Those who travelled to Europe and the United States brought home with them new ideas and fashions. While the tribal rulers did their best to uphold tradition, the Western-educated few were regarded as trend-setting members of society, apostles of a new order. Less privileged citizens began to emulate them. Change was in motion: old customs started to give way to new alternatives. Among other indicators of change, hairdressers in modernized urban areas erected signs declaring that they were London- or Paris-trained.

These developments in Africa coincided with the rise of the civil rights movement in the United States. Black Americans who had ignored their cultural past or had been

51
Nigerian Independence celebrations at St. Anne's School, Ibadan, October 1960. HRH Princess Alexandra watching a student's demonstration of cornrowing and hair threading.

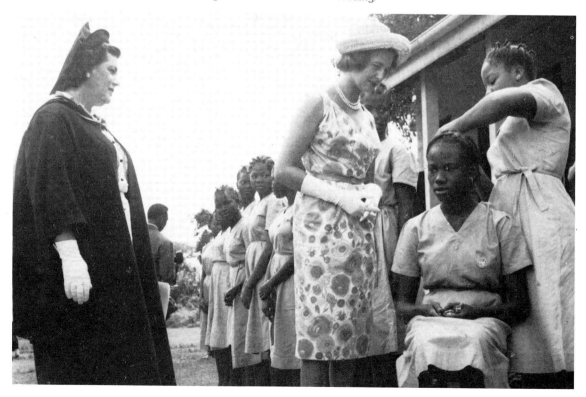

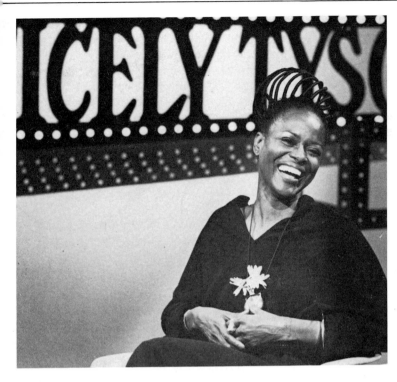

52
Cicely Tyson on the Mike Douglas Show in America wearing her hair threaded in the *Eko Bridge* style.

denied access to it were intently searching for roots, for something African with which to identify. African performers such as Babatunde Olatunji of Nigeria and Miriam Makeba of South Africa stirred Black consciousness in the United States with their music, dances and fashion. Blacks all over the North American continent vibrated with a new sense of awareness and with racial pride, which was evident in their adoption of African fashions and the afro hairstyle. (Although the afro was for some time symbolic of Black militancy, it soon became generally fashionable.)

After the afro came the cornrowing craze. Cornrowing had been known among Blacks ever since their arrival in the United States, but those who had worn their hair in that style had always concealed it under wigs or kerchiefs. Fearing that the style would not be accepted by the white establishment, Blacks had never dared to display it publicly. Braiding and cornrowing were considered acceptable for children but unbecoming on adults. A few years ago, however, the actress Cicely Tyson helped to change this attitude by wearing her hair cornrowed on television (**52**). She startled the nation, but the style captured the imagination of culture-conscious Blacks, who put aside their wigs and processed hair to try out the technique for themselves. Cornrowing spread across the United States like wildfire and is now worn by young men and women alike.

Now that independence has been attained by most African countries, there has been a general resurgence of interest in African culture, and a conscious effort is being made to preserve those indigenous styles and techniques of every craft that have survived.

It is refreshing to see that traditional hairdressers – who have held their ground during this half-century of change – are very much in vogue in large cities and towns in Africa. West Africans in particular have done a great deal to revive and experiment with cornrowing and hair threading techniques and to confer on them the status of high fashion. Travel and the communication media have helped to spread traditional styles and techniques across the globe and have drawn together the entire Black world. Hairstyles that were once considered the mark of priesthood, royalty or ethnic tradition now have general appeal.

Cornrowing

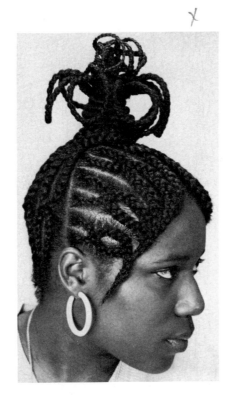

Cornrowing

Cornrowing is braiding or plaiting. The technique, in which the hair is braided firmly on the surface of the scalp, depends for its effect on the patterns, simple or intricate, that are formed on the scalp by the parting of the hair.

In recent years there have been countless innovations in cornrowing that it is almost impossible to name each new style. There are however traditional Yoruba names for basic styles such as *Suku*, basket (**53**); *Ipako Elede*, occiput of a pig (**54**); *Koroba*, bucket (**55**) and *Kolese*, without legs (**56**).

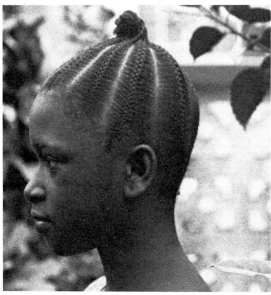

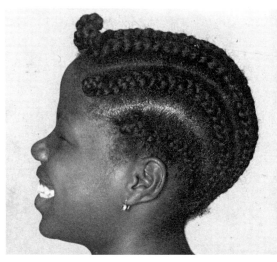

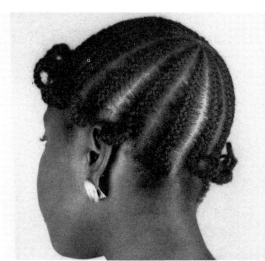

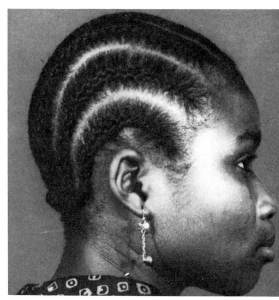

How to cornrow

The basic requirements are a comb and any kind of hair grease or hair oil.

There are two methods of cornrowing, which result in slightly different types of braid. One method is to braid with an *overhand* motion, sometimes known as 'right-side' cornrowing (**57**); the other is to braid with an *underhand* motion, known as 'wrong-side' cornrowing (**58**). The underhand method appears to be the more popular today.

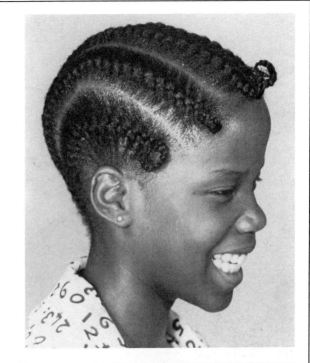

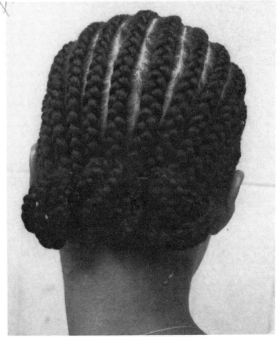

53 *opposite top left*
Suku

54 *opposite top right*
Ipako Elede

55 *opposite bottom left*
Koroba

56 *opposite bottom right*
Kolese

57 *top right*
Inverted cornrowing, sometimes known as 'right-side' cornrowing, done with an overhand motion.

58 *bottom right*
'Wrong-side' cornrowing which results from braiding with an underhand motion.

For beginners it is best to experiment on medium-length hair at 3-4 inches (75-100 millimetres) long. A simple, traditional six-sectioned style like *Ipako Elede* (**59**) provides an opportunity to practise the rudiments of cornrowing.

1 Comb the hair to straighten out tight, kinky curls.
2 Make a centre parting from the front of the hairline to the nape of the neck, and secure one half of the parted hair with a comb, clips or a rubber band.
3 Part the other half of the hair into three equal longitudinal sections.

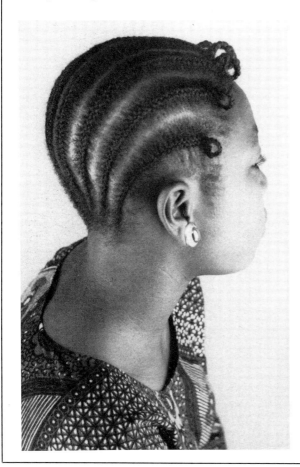

4 Oil each section.
5 Starting with the section furthest from the top of the head and *working from the back of the head towards the front*, take three small portions of hair and braid them firmly into a threefold strand that lies flat on the scalp.
6 Continue to cornrow by picking up hair from the roots at short intervals and weaving it into each strand.
7 At the front of the head braid the hair to the very tip and twist to give the ends a tidy finish.
8 Repeat the process on the second and third rows, making your way up to the top of the head.
9 Cornrow the other half of the hair using the same method.

To keep the style neat, wrap the head with a scarf at bedtime. Oil the scalp thoroughly every day to avoid dandruff. Although some styles last for two or three weeks, it is best to undo the braids and wash the hair about once a week.

One advantage of cornrowing the hair regularly is that it makes the hair grow thick and long.

59
The traditional six-sectioned style, *Ipako Elede*.

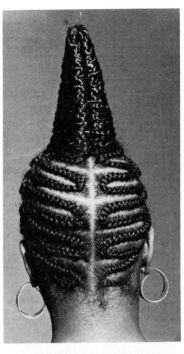

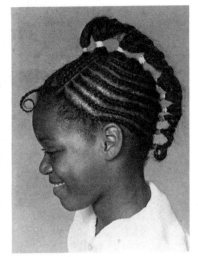

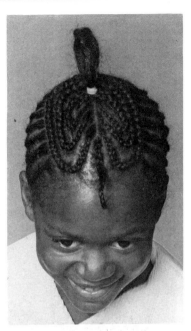

60 a & b *top and bottom left*
The hair is divided into four sections lengthwise and crosswise. Each section is then braided to give this snakey effect. For added height a braided cone-shaped hairpiece is attached to the top.

61 a & b *above and top right*
At the front a small 'A' shape is parted and braided. The remaining front section is parted into a horseshoe shape, divided into two equal parts and then sectioned into six strips crosswise. These are braided upwards and held in a rubber band. The hair is then parted from the crown to the nape and seven strips on each side are braided to the back of the head. The remainder of the hair on top of the head is parted into several cross strips and braided. All the loose ends meeting in the middle are secured with rubber bands and lightly braided into one row.

62 *bottom right*
Both sides are coiled. The centre is parted and braided into circles while the front and back are braided away from the crown.

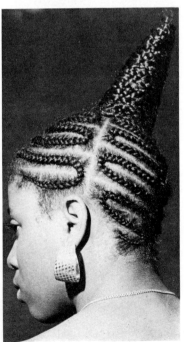

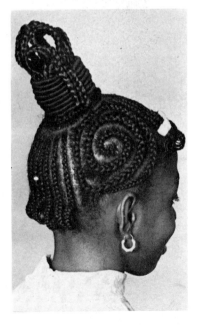

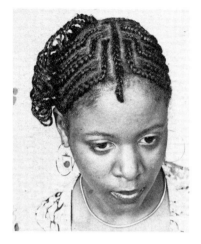

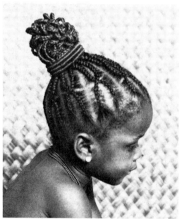

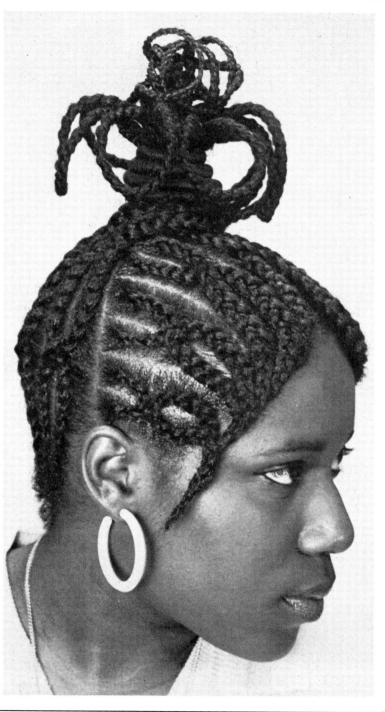

63 *top left*
A thin centre strip is braided forward. One front section is then braided to the right and ends just behind the ear. The left section is braided all the way round the back of the head to the right side and neatly arranged into braided curls.

64 *bottom left*
An unusual style of cornrowing called chainbraiding which results in a series of Xs. The hair is parted and braided into eighteen strips beginning from the hairline and ending at the crown. A hairpiece is then attached at the top.

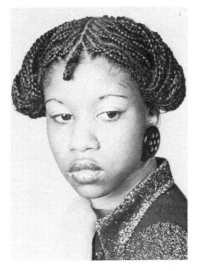
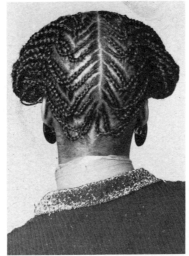
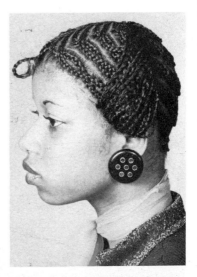

65 *opposite right*
The front is parted and braided forward into rows of Xs. The ends are carefully connected and arranged on either side of the face. The back is braided upwards and the ends tucked into a hairpiece.

66 a, b & c *top left, middle and right*
Another example of chainbraiding.

67 *bottom right*
Combined chainbraiding and plain cornrowing. Every other row is chainbraided upwards and the rows cornrowed downwards are arranged in flat curls at the ends. The braids meeting at the top of the head are neatly connected and decorated with beads.

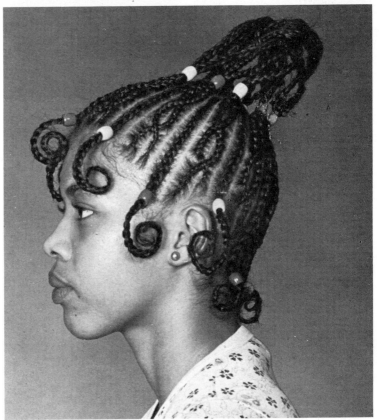

55

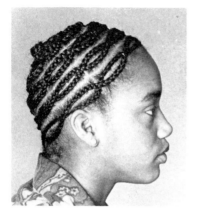

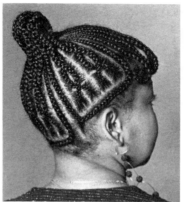

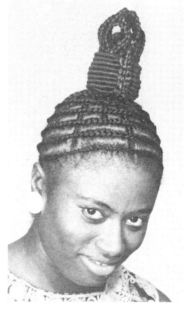

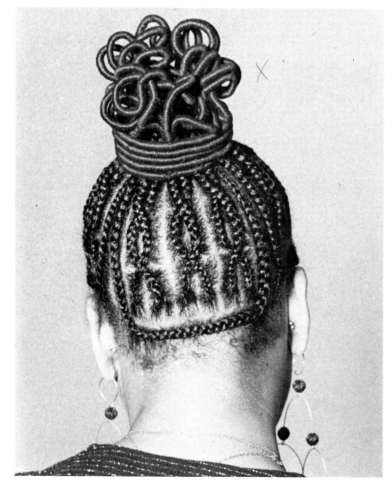

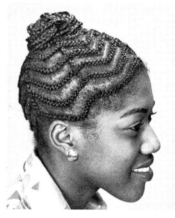

68 *top left*
Beginning from the bottom left of the head, the chainbraid is one continuous row going round and round and ending at the top of the head.

69 a & b *top middle and bottom left*
Combined chainbraiding and plain cornrowing. **69b** shows the style with an added hairpiece.

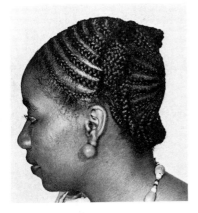

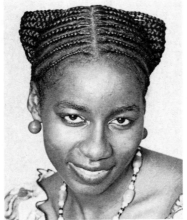

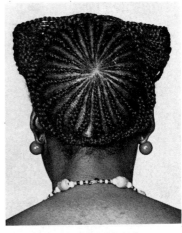

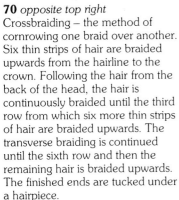

70 *opposite top right*
Crossbraiding – the method of cornrowing one braid over another. Six thin strips of hair are braided upwards from the hairline to the crown. Following the hair from the back of the head, the hair is continuously braided until the third row from which six more thin strips of hair are braided upwards. The transverse braiding is continued until the sixth row and then the remaining hair is braided upwards. The finished ends are tucked under a hairpiece.

71 *opposite bottom right*
The hair is crossbraided as in **70** except that the transverse braids form a series of zig-zags.

72 a, b & c *top left, middle and right*
Starting just behind the ears, the hair is parted across the top of the head. The front section is then divided in two from the crown to the forehead. Each half is sectioned and braided back in thin strips. The radial effect at the back is achieved by dividing the hair into twenty-two strips and braiding it outwards from the back of the head. At either side all the ends are neatly attached together.

73 *bottom right*
Cornrowing and chainbraiding.

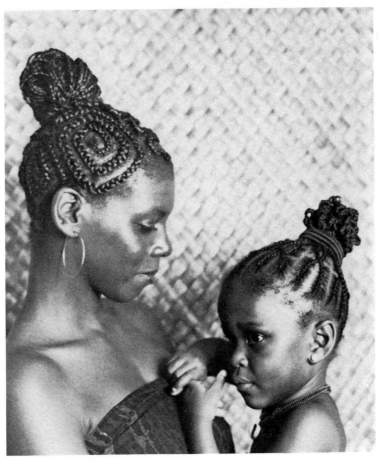

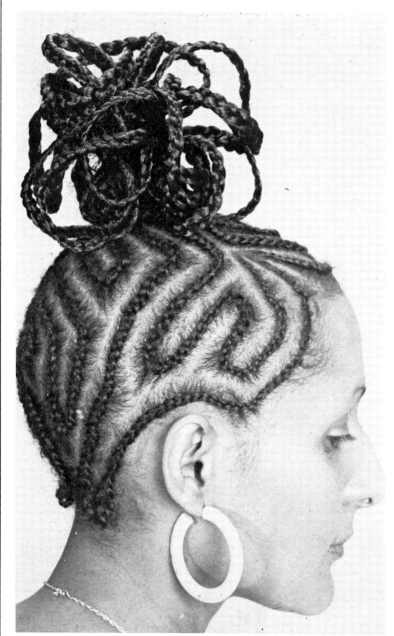

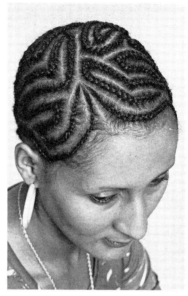

74 a & b *above and left*
Starting from the front and ending at the nape of the neck, the braids meander over the entire head. A hairpiece is then attached to the crown.

75 a, b, c & d *opposite*
Each side is divided into thirteen strips and braided to form a star and the ends are curled. The front section is braided upwards forming four 'U' shapes and the braids at the back meander upwards ending at the crown.

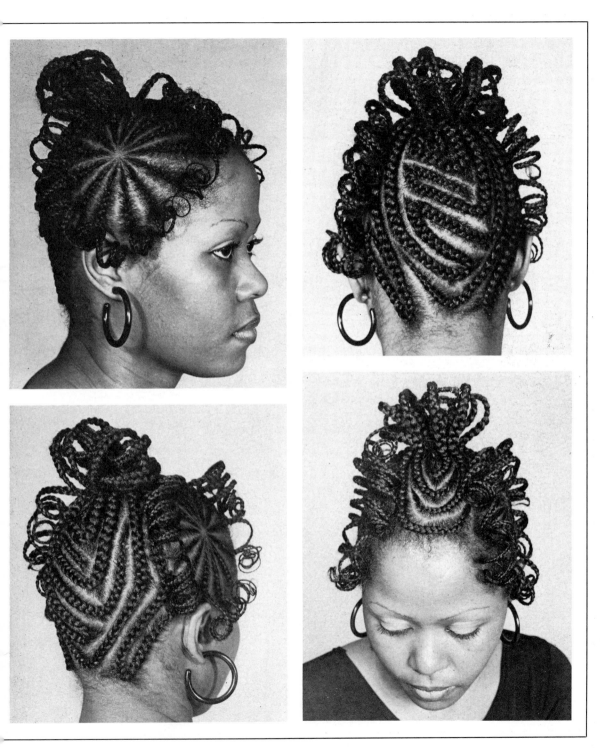

Cornrowing with an attachment

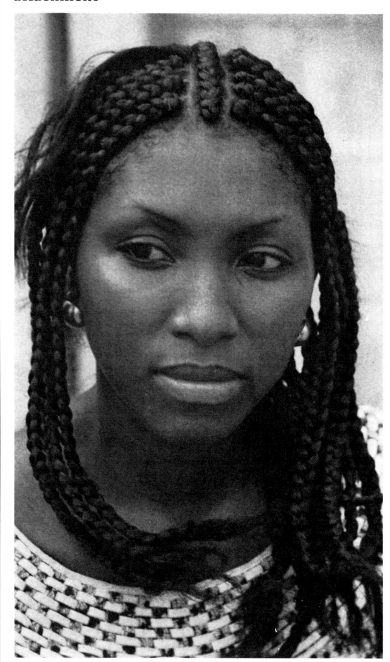

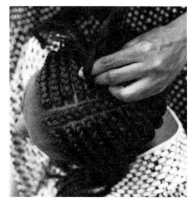

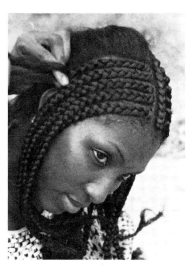

76 *this page and opposite*
This series of pictures shows how to cornrow with an attachment (also known as weaving).
a) notice the length and thickness of the false hairpiece.
b & c) the hairdresser attaches the hairpiece to the scalp and begins to cornrow.
d) once the cornrowing is finished the hairdresser stitches the ends of the braids together using a needle and black thread.
e) the ends are then rolled up and stitched into position.

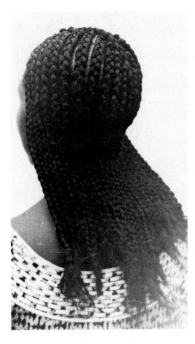

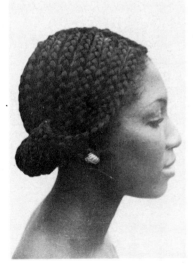

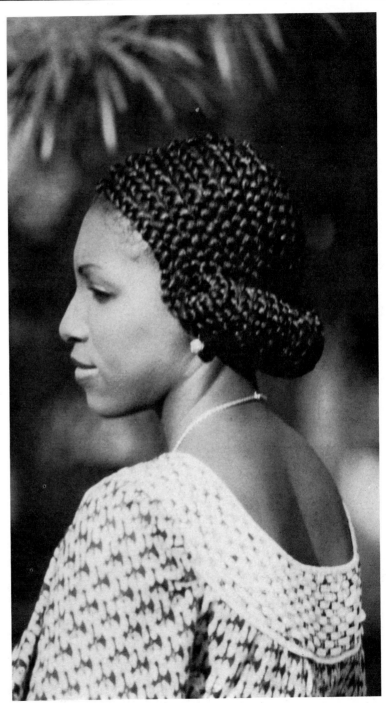

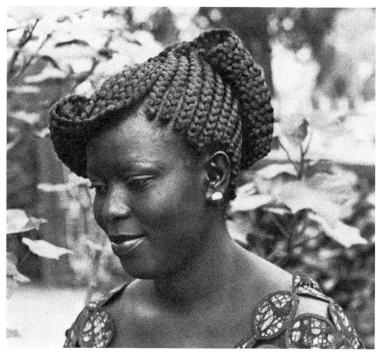

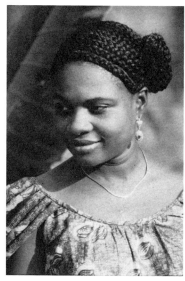

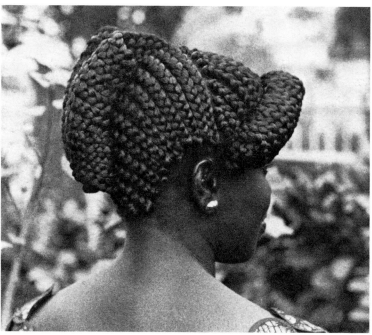

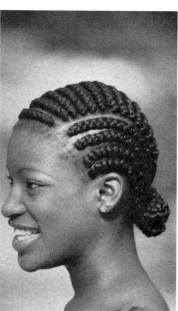

77-80
Cornrowing with an attachment.

Men's styles

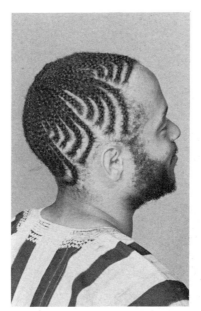
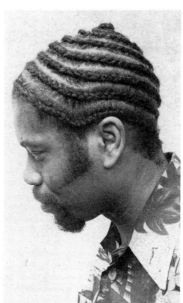

81 *top right*
Cornrowed styles on men should follow the contours of the head to fit like a cap. The hair is parted into eight sections from the crown. Each section is divided into five 'J' strips and braided upwards, the ends connecting neatly at the top.

82 *top far right*
Beginning from the bottom right of the head, the hair is braided in one continuous circle ending at the top.

83 a & b *bottom left and right*
In this style the hair has been braided into four circles.

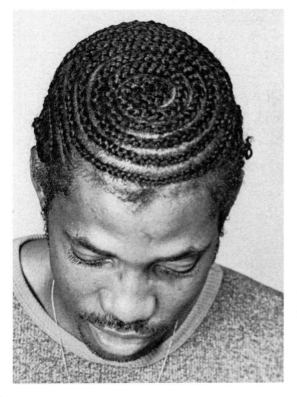
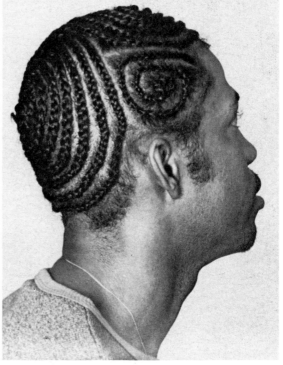

Hair Threading

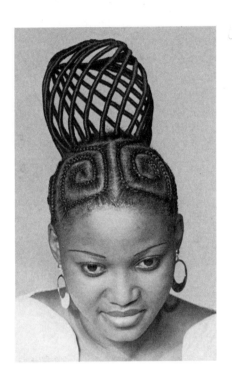

Hair threading is a recently coined term for the technique of wrapping sectioned hair with black thread. All the styles are three-dimensional and are a combination of a) patterns etched on the scalp and b) threaded strands which are raised from the scalp.

Southern Nigeria, where the technique is highly developed, has provided names for many of the styles of threaded hair: *Kudeti* (an area in Ibadan township where the oldest girls' school was situated); *Los* (an abbreviation for Los Angeles, where Nigeria's former featherweight boxing champion, Hogan Kid-Bassey, won his title in the late 1950s); *Eko Bridge* (a modern bridge in Lagos, Nigeria's capital city); *Sungas* (a type of cooking gas); *Air Force* (a style that evolved during the Nigerian Civil War); *Akula* ('Don't touch: he is crazy!'); *Sinkro System* (a type of dance).

As in cornrowing a number of things are taken into consideration before beginning to thread, such as: the length of hair, the design on the scalp and the design on the threaded strands. The length of hair is mainly what determines the simplicity or complexity of the style. For short hair, anything between 1-2 inches, styles are very limited. Long hair is always an advantage because it lends itself to numerous and more elaborate styles.

The design parted on the scalp

There is an endless range of scalp designs formed by parting the hair lengthwise, crosswise, or into curves. The basic designs are: *Star* (**85**), *Crown* (**86**), *Pineapple* (**87**) and *Kudeti* (**88**).

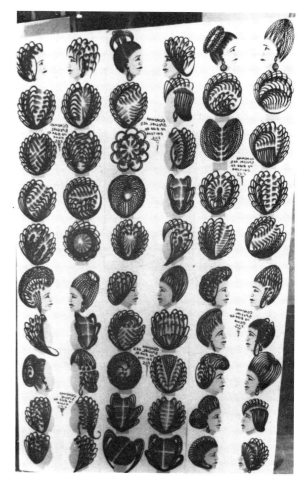

84 *above*
Signboard in front of local hairdresser's store.

85 *opposite top left*
Star

86 *opposite top right*
Crown

87 *opposite bottom left*
Pineapple

88 *opposite bottom right*
Kudeti

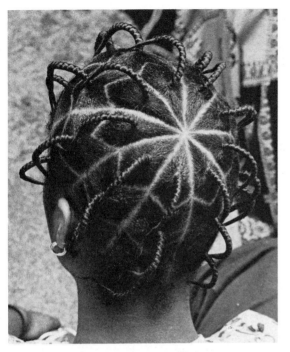
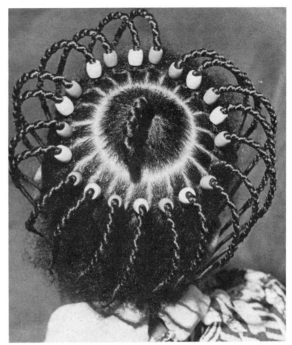
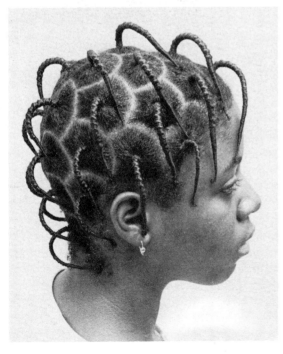
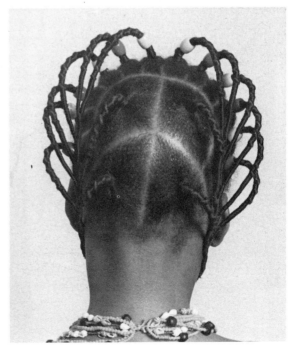

The design on threaded strands

These are designs created on the strands of hair as a result of twisting or varying the spaces between wrapped hair. The basic designs are shown in illustrations **89-97**.

1 *Onigi* (**89**). This is the original way the hair was threaded before later hairdressers introduced new variations. In Yoruba *onigi* means sticks, so called because of the way the threaded strands of hair are left standing on end all over the head. To achieve this effect, thread is wrapped around the base of a section of loose hair four or five times and then wrapping is continued to the end of the hair. The thread is then tied and the extra length is cut off.

2 *Okoto* or *Puff* (**90**). A section of hair is threaded for about a quarter-of-an-inch from the scalp. The hair is twisted anti-clockwise and a section left unthreaded. As the thread is wound round the hair below the unthreaded space, it is pulled tight, as if gathering, and this creates the *Puff*. The rest of the hair is then threaded to the end. For more elaborate designs several *Puffs* can be made along the same length of hair and this is then called *Quadrupled Okoto* (four *Puffs* on one section) or *Multiple Okoto*.

3 *Dada* (**91**) (a Yoruba word applied to children born with naturally matted hair). This style is a combination of the braiding and threading techniques. After the hair at the scalp has been wrapped with thread a few times, the hair is braided away from the scalp for about half its length. The rest of the hair is then threaded to the end.

4 *Sungas* (**92**). The hair is twisted anticlockwise before threading and is threaded in such a manner that no hair shows.

5 *Bubbled Sungas* (**93**). This is slightly different from Sungas in that the threaded strands are interspersed with tiny bubbles. The hair is twisted anti-clockwise and threaded a quarter-of-an-inch away from the base. Then the individual bubbles are created after every three very close wraps which gives the style a scalloped effect.

6 *Ejo* (**94**) (the Yoruba word for snake). As for *Sungas*, the hair is twisted anticlockwise, then threaded closely from the scalp to the ends of the hair. To achieve the snake-like effect, the hair is wound around a pencil four or five times.

7 *Twist* (**95**). Half an inch of hair is wrapped at the base and then the loose hair is separated into two equal portions. The strands are twisted anticlockwise, threaded individually, intertwined and then tied at the end.

8 *Sulphur 8* (**96**). This strand design is named after a particular type of hair pomade known as 'Sulphur 8'. A section of hair is first threaded into the *Sungas* design leaving about 6 inches of thread at the tip. The fully threaded bunch of hair is then twisted to form the figure 8 and the remaining thread at the tip is wrapped round the base several times and tied.

9 *Koso* (**97**). In this design the hair is also threaded into the *Sungas* design leaving thread at the end of the hair. The fully threaded strand is then bent downwards and twisted around the base three or four times. The thread is then tied securely round the base a few times and cut off.

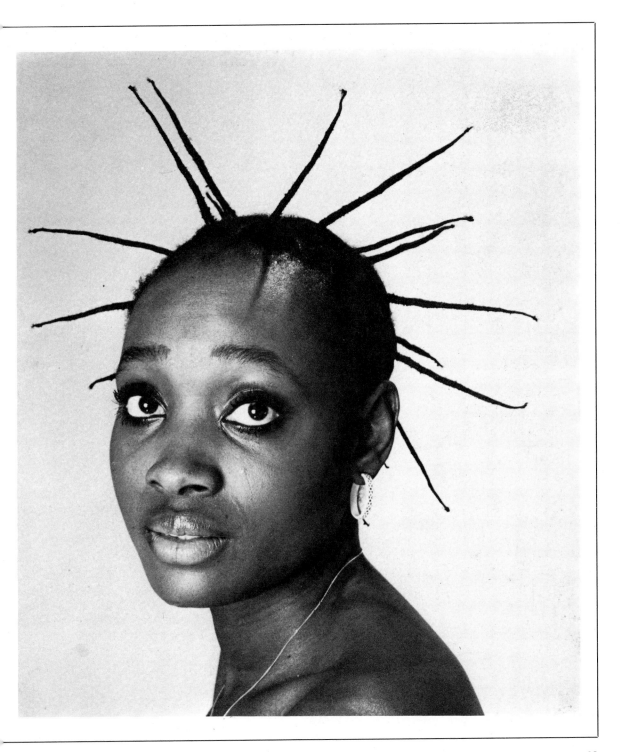

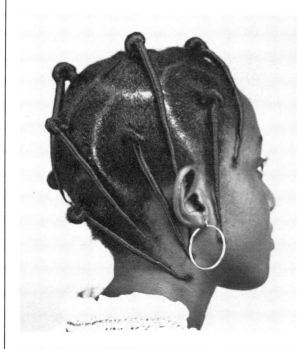

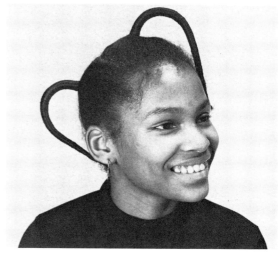

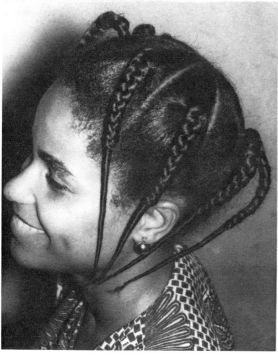

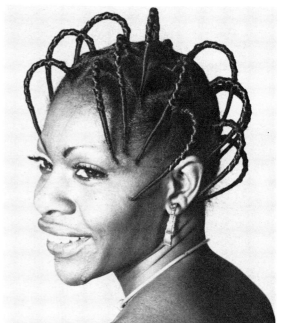

89 *page 69*
Onigi

90 *top left*
Okoto or Puff

91 *bottom left*
Dada

92 *top right*
Sungas

93 *bottom right*
Bubbled Sungas

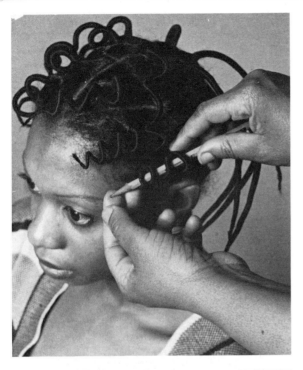

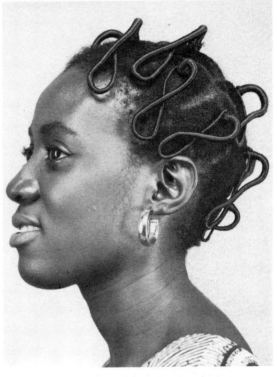

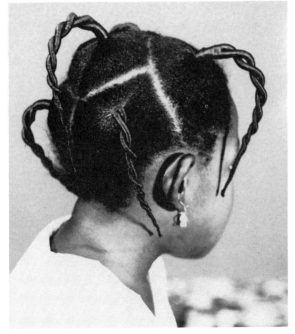

94 *top left*
Ejo or *Snake*

95 *bottom left*
The Twist

96 *top right*
Sulphur 8

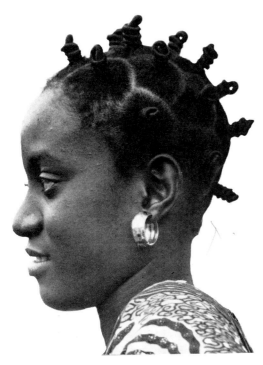

97 *above*
Koso

How to thread hair

The basic requirements are a comb (preferably a four- or five-pronged wooden one), hair grease, a razor blade or a pair of scissors and spools of black thread (cotton or man-made).

Beginners should practise threading on long hair (7-8 inches; 180-200 millimetres), which can be sectioned into three or four parts. It is important to wrap the hair evenly and to guard against scalp tension, caused by pulling the hair in wrapping it too tightly. *Onigi* (sticks) is a simple style on which to experiment.

1 Comb the hair to straighten out tight, kinky curls.
2 Divide the hair into 16 sections.
3 Using clips or rubber bands, secure each of the sections of hair except the one on which you plan to work first.
4 Oil the section that you are about to thread.
5 Taking about 1 yard (approximately 1 metre) of doubled or quadrupled black thread in your right hand, hold the oiled section of hair firmly at the scalp between your left thumb and forefinger.
6 Having anchored the end of the thread by twisting it around the hair at the scalp, wind the thread clockwise around the section of hair, working your way gradually towards the hair ends.
7 When you reach the tip of the hair ends, knot the thread securely two or three times so that it does not unravel.
8 Cut off the end of the thread with a pair of scissors or a razor blade.

9 Repeat the same process with each of the parted sections until all of the hair has been threaded.

To keep the hair neat, wrap the head with a scarf at bedtime. (Sleeping on threaded hair is no more uncomfortable than sleeping on rollers.) Oil the scalp thoroughly every day to avoid dandruff. Hair can remain threaded for about a week, after which it should be unwrapped and washed.

Threading encourages the hair to grow faster because of the traction, but constant threading has a tendency to make the hairline recede, especially from the temples. It is advisable, therefore, to alternate between cornrowing and threading from time to time.

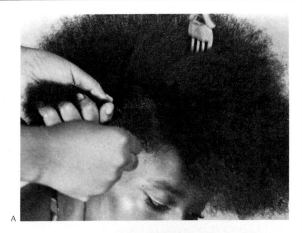

A

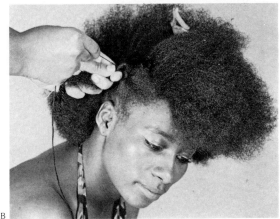

B

98 a-g
These pictures show how to thread the *Okoto* style.
a) a section of hair is parted and held firmly between the left thumb and forefinger and the threading begins.
b) after threading the base, the hair is pulled into a big 'bubble' shape known as 'okoto'.
c) the threading continues along the length of the hair.

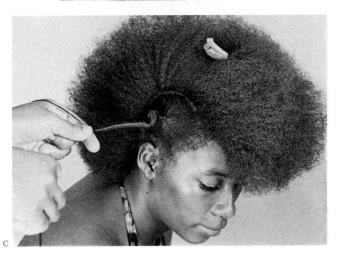

C

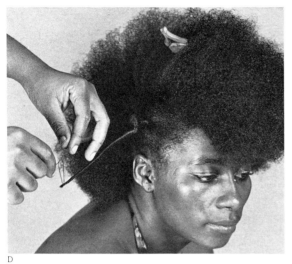

D

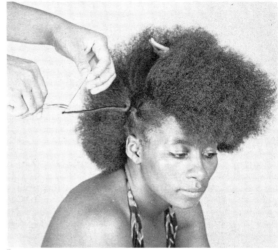

E

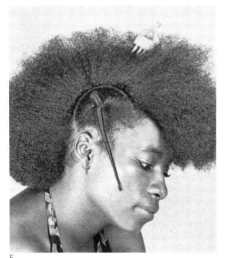

F

d) the thread is tied several times round the end of the hair to stop it unravelling.

e) the thread is cut.

f) the completed bunch of hair.

g) the finished hairstyle.

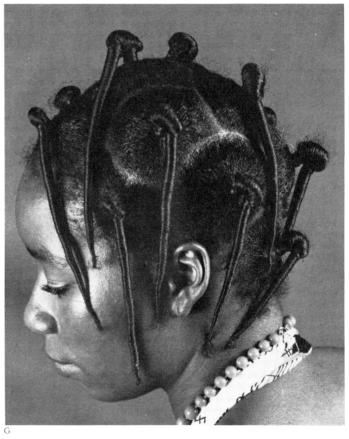

G

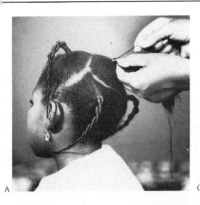

A

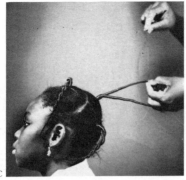

C

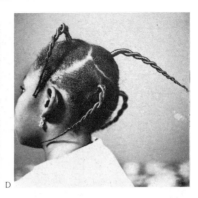

D

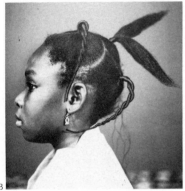

B

99 a-e

How to thread the *Twist*.

a) about half an inch of hair is threaded at the base.

b) the loose hair is then divided into two equal parts.

c) each section of hair is twisted anti-clockwise and then threaded individually.

d) to achieve the twisted effect the two threaded strands are intertwined, wrapped at the tail-end and bent downwards.

e) the finished hairstyle.

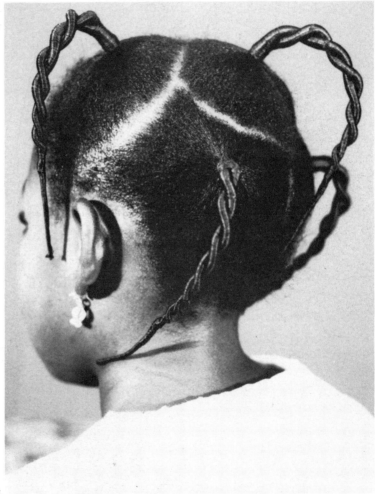

E

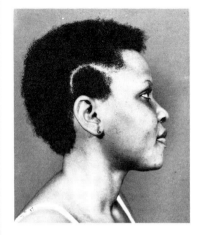
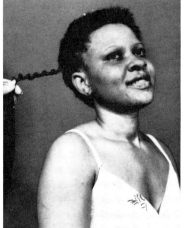
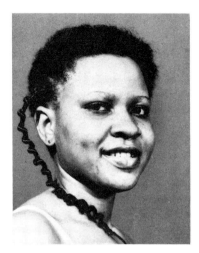
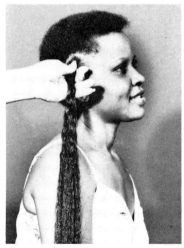
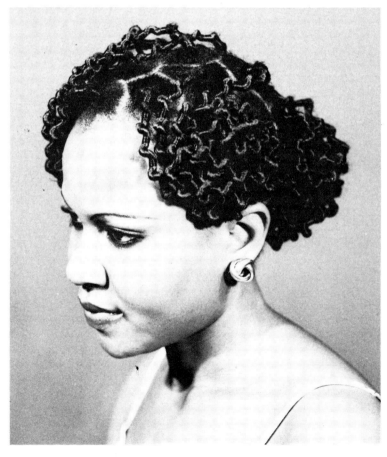

100 a-e

How to thread the multiple *Okoto* on short hair.

a) a small section of hair is parted into a curve and oiled.

b) a hairpiece is attached to the hair from the scalp.

c) the hairpiece is threaded in the multiple *Okoto* design.

d) finished section.

e) threaded into thirty sections, the ends are connected and arranged into three bunches of curls, one at each side and one at the back.

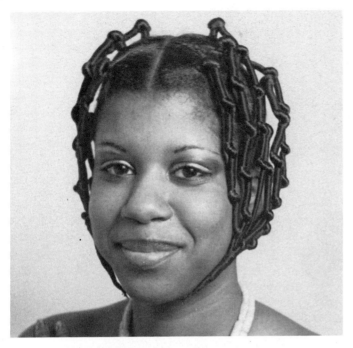

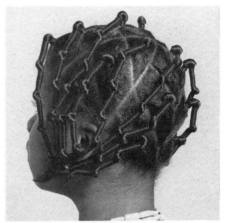

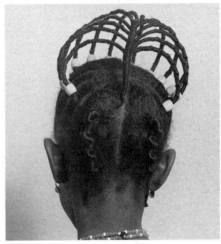

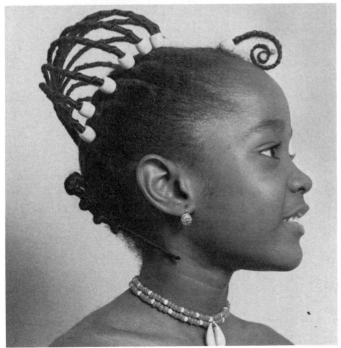

101 a & b *top left and right*
Parted into eighteen sections the hair is threaded in the multiple *Okoto* design and connected into two bunches, one on each side of the face.

102 a & b *bottom left and right*
This style combines three designs. The hair is parted into fifteen sections. At the front a small spiral plait is made, standing away from the head. The central section is threaded into the *Bubbled Sungas* design using wool, wire and beads. The ends are connected to form a coronet. The back is threaded in the quadrupled *Okoto* design.

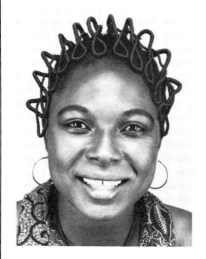

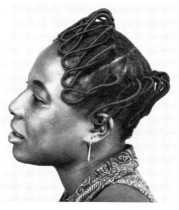

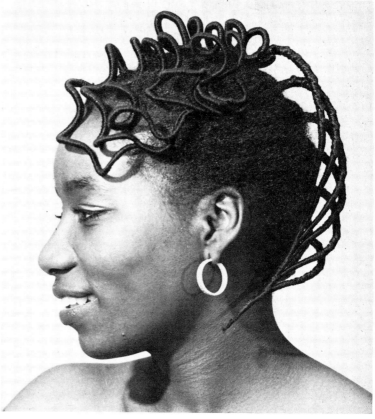

103 a, b & c *top, middle and bottom left*
Sulphur 8 design threaded into twenty-one parts.

104 a & b *top and bottom right*
Nineteen sections are threaded in a combination of the *Snake* and *Bubbled Sungas* designs.

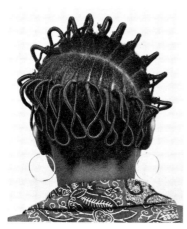

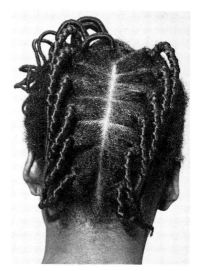

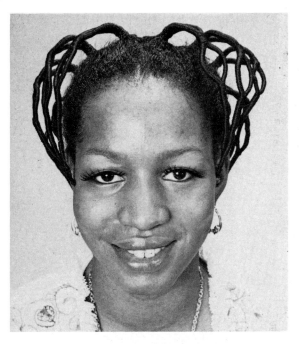

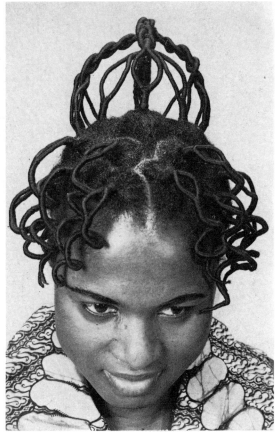

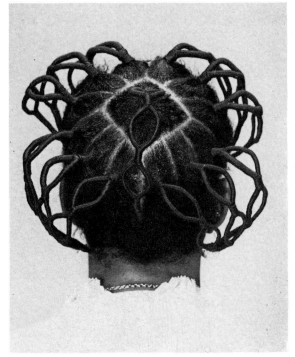

105 a & b *top and bottom left*
Parted into thirteen, the hair is
threaded into a series of 'eyelets'.
This is achieved by threading a
section of hair about a quarter of an
inch from the base. The hair is then
divided into two, threaded
separately for an inch or more and
then joined and threaded together
for half an inch. This process is then
repeated forming another 'eyelet'
and then threaded to the end. The
ends are then grouped in threes
and point towards the neck.

106 *above*
The 'eyelet' (as shown in **105**) and
Snake designs are combined here.

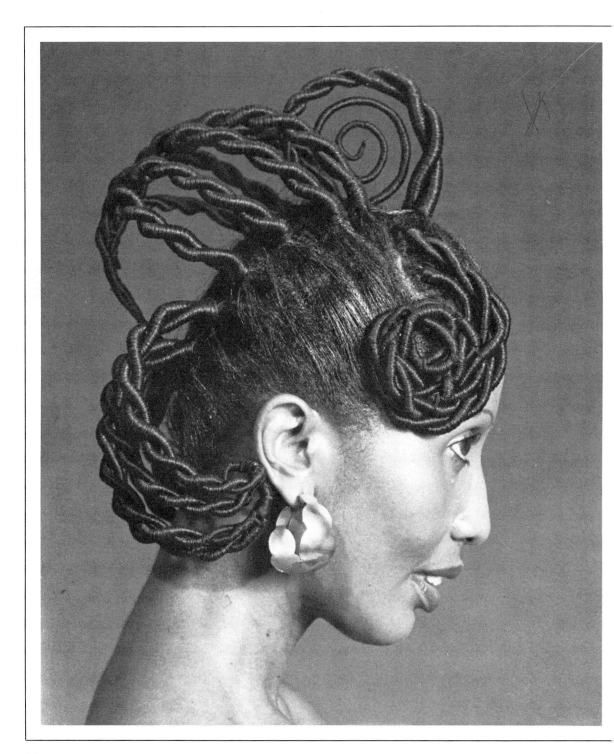

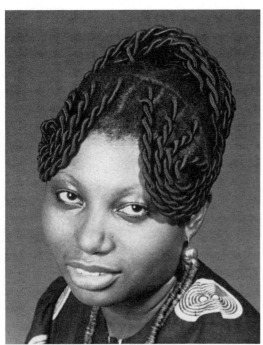

107 *opposite*
The hair is parted in twenty-four sections and threaded in the *Twist* design.

108 a & b *top and bottom left*
A variation of the *Twist*. The hair is threaded in the *Onigi* design and arranged into twists. The front is sectioned into eight strands on each side, twisted in twos and the back is parted into twenty-four, threaded and also twisted in twos.

109 *below*
This style is called *Eko Bridge*. The hair is parted into twenty-four sections forming a star at the centre of the head. Each strand is then threaded in the *Onigi* design and the tips of each strand are connected until they form a circle.

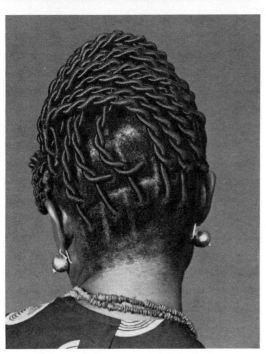

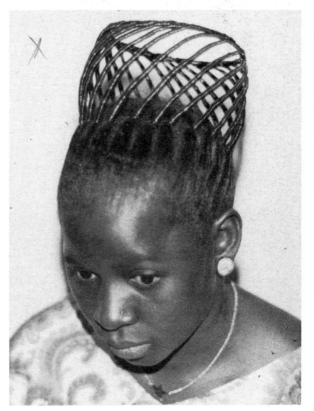

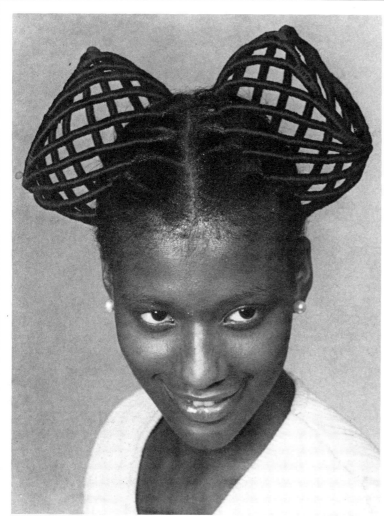

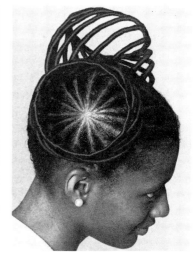

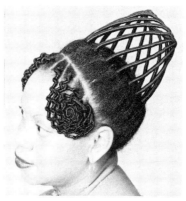

110 a & b *above and top right*
Each side is parted into fifteen
sections and the strands are
threaded to form two *Eko Bridges*,
one on each side of the head and
set at an angle to each other.

111 *middle right*
The *Eko Bridge* design is combined
with multiple *Okoto* formed into
rosettes on either side of the face.

112 *bottom right*
This style combines the *Eko Bridge*
and *Sulphur 8* designs.

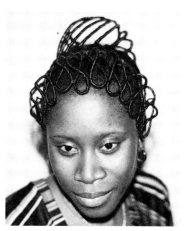

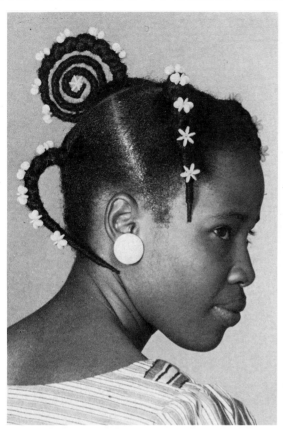

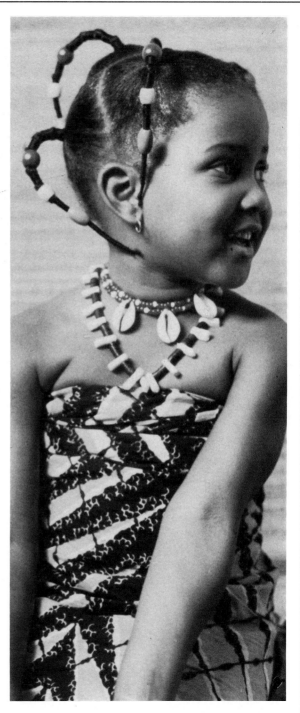

113 *above*
Divided into four sections the strands are threaded in the *Bubbled Sungas* design. Using wool and some copper wire the hair is coiled upright on the crown. Artificial flowers are used for decoration.

114 *right*
Showing the hairstyle on a child, the hair is parted into five sections, threaded in *Bubbled Sungas* and decorated with beads.

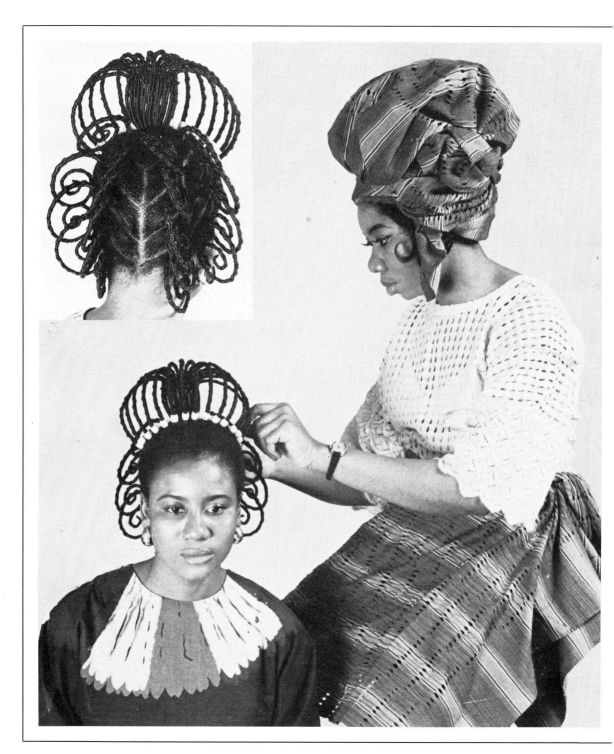

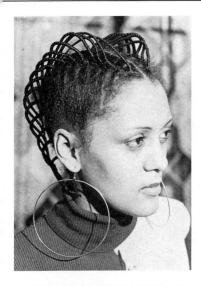

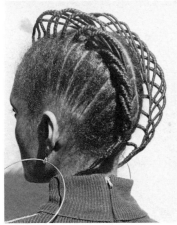

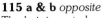

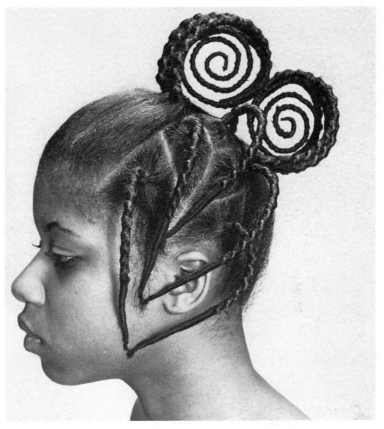

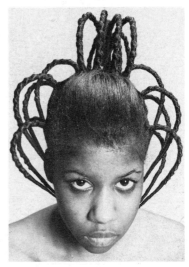

115 a & b *opposite*
The hair is parted across the top of the head from ear to ear. The front section is sectioned into fourteen parts which are beaded, threaded in the *Bubbled Sungas* design and arranged into a crown with the ends sewn together. Using wool and copper wire, the back section is divided into sixteen and also threaded into the *Bubbled Sungas* design. These threaded strips are then curled.

116 a & b *top and bottom left*
To achieve this style, the hair is parted down the middle of the head and each half is divided into fifteen sections. Each section is threaded in the *Bubbled Sungas* design and connected on each side in a pattern resembling cross hatching.

117 a & b *above and bottom right*
Another variation of the *Bubbled Sungas* design.

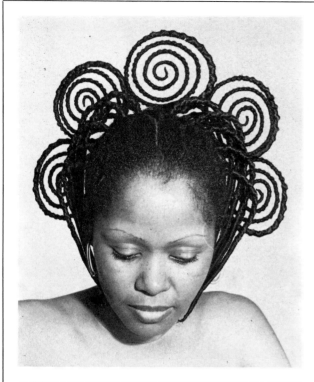

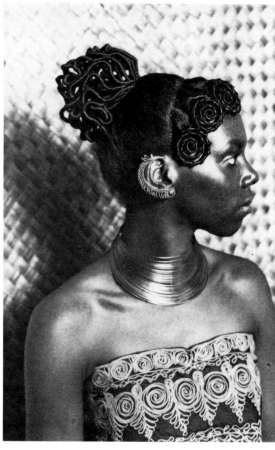

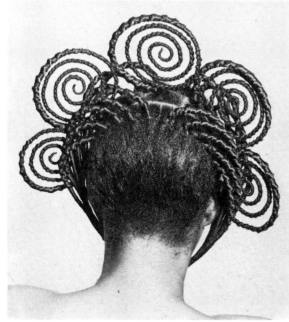

118 *above*
A style combining two designs. The front is threaded in the *Bubbled Sungas* design and arranged in flat curls on the forehead whilst the hair at the back is fastened together and covered by a hairpiece threaded in the *Snake* design.

119 a & b *top and bottom left*
This style requires very long hair. At the front, five sections on each side are threaded in the *Bubbled Sungas* design and connected. This is then repeated with the hair at the back of the head. The hair on the top of the head is then threaded and made into five upright coils.

120 a & b *top right and far right*
A section of hair on the top of the head is threaded into a large spiral using wool and wire. The remaining hair is parted vertically into twenty-two sections, each is individually wired, threaded in the *Bubbled Sungas* design and curled.

121 a & b *bottom left and right*
Using the *Bubbled Sungas* design the hair is arranged into flat ringlets on the forehead and made into a 'coronet' on the top of the head.

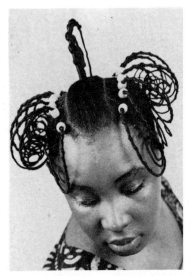
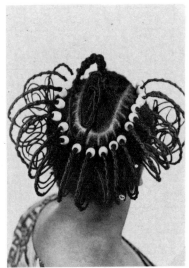
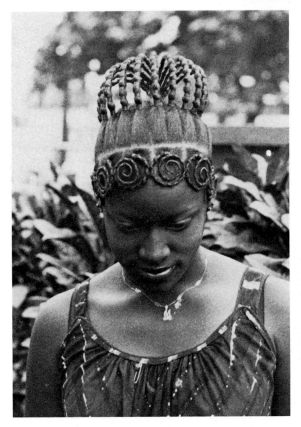
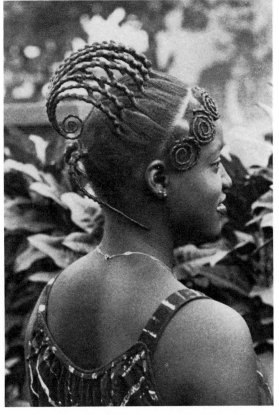

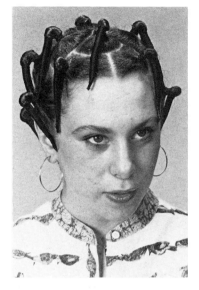

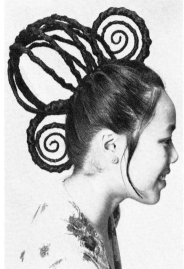

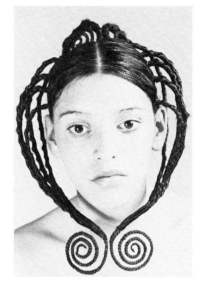

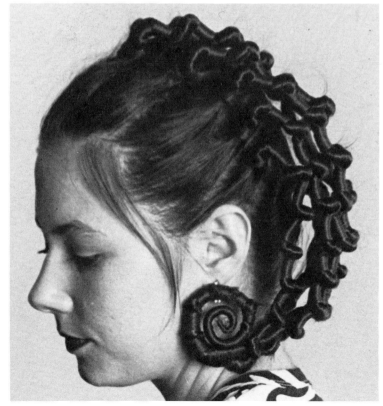

Caucasian & Oriental hairstyles

122 *top left*
Caucasian hair parted into ten sections and threaded in the single *Okoto* design.

123 *top middle*
The hair is parted into ten sections and threaded in the *Bubbled Sungas* design.

124 *top right*
The *Bubbled Sungas* design is combined with the coil or spiral motif.

125 *bottom left*
The hair is threaded in the multiple *Okoto* design, coiled at the end.

126 *opposite*
The multiple *Okoto* design again on Caucasian hair.

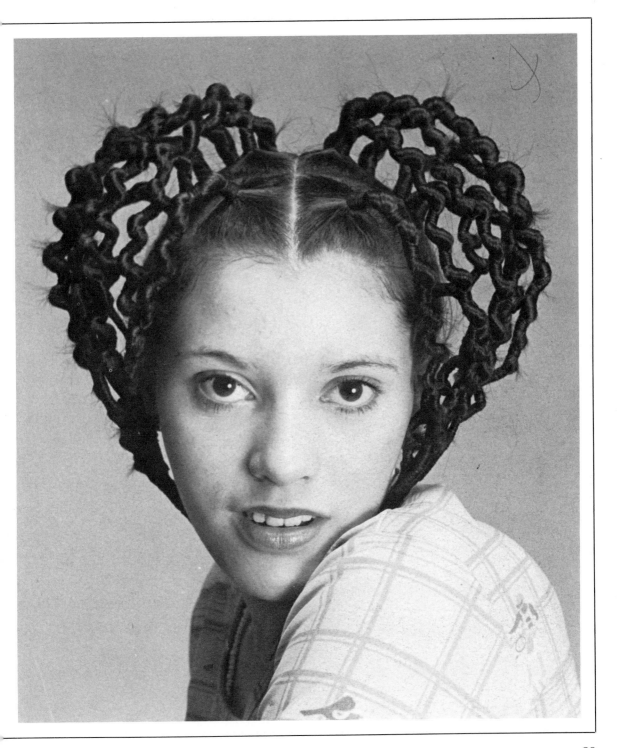

Combined Cornrowing
& Hair Threading

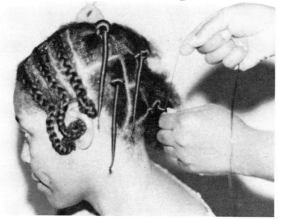

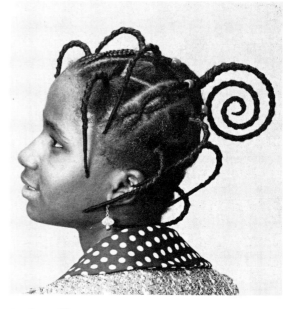

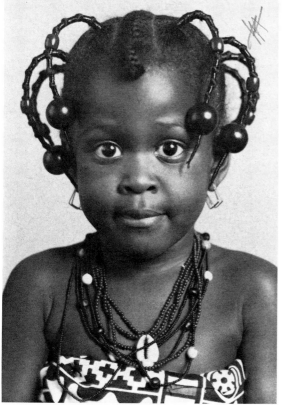

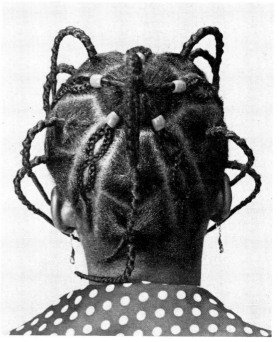

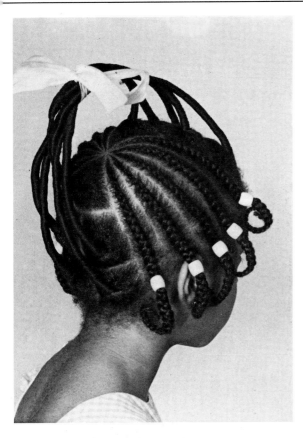

130 a & b *left and below*
The front and back sections of hair are parted in an 'A' shape. Each is then divided into five, threaded in the *Onigi* design and connected at the top. Each side is parted, braided downwards and beads are slipped through the ends which are twisted into curls.

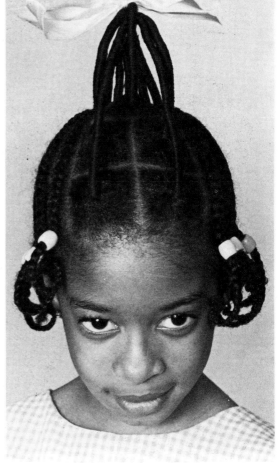

127 *opposite top left*
Combined cornrowing and hair threading.

128 a & b *opposite top and bottom right*
The *Bubbled Sungas* design is combined with chainbraiding.

129 *opposite bottom left*
The central strip of hair is braided using the 'right-side' method of cornrowing while the rest is threaded in the *Bubbled Sungas* design.

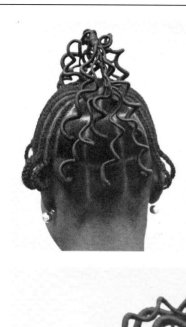

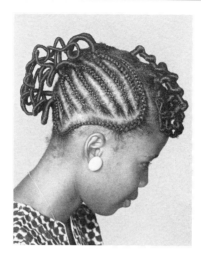

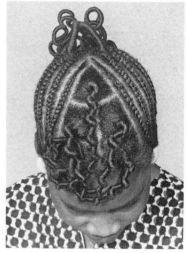

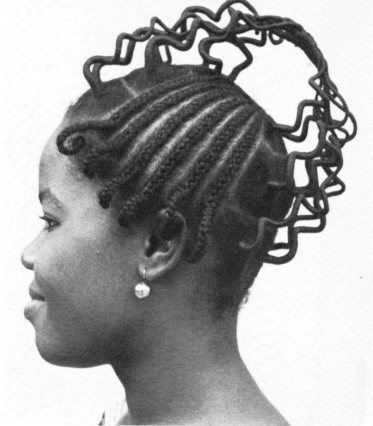

131 a & b *top and bottom left*
A combination of inverted cornrowing and the *Snake* method of threading.

132 a & b *top middle and right*
This hairstyle combines cornrowing with hair threaded in both the multiple *Okoto* and *Snake* designs.

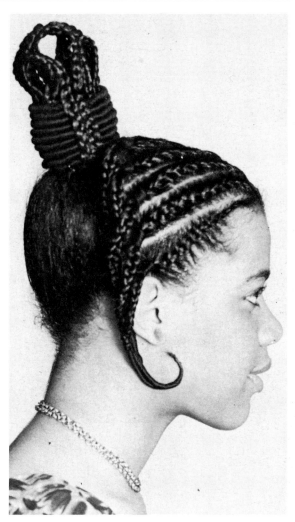

133 a & b
The hair at the front is braided
away from the centre in five rows
on each side and the ends are then
threaded in the *Dada* design. The
back section of hair is drawn
together on top of the head and
neatly covered by a hairpiece that is
partly threaded and partly braided.

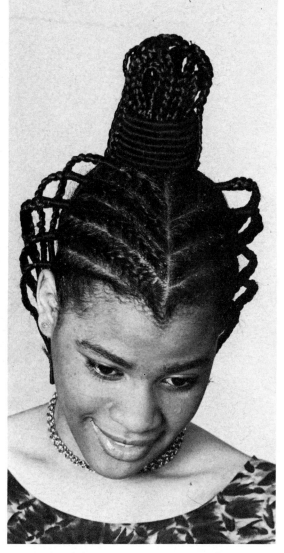

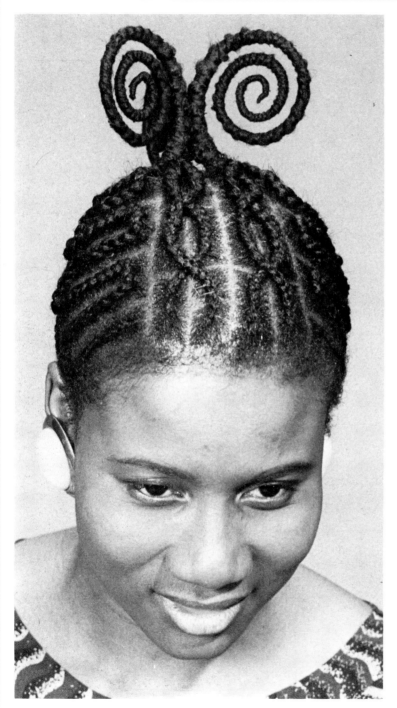
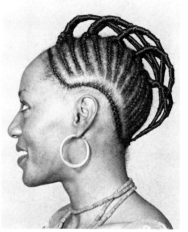
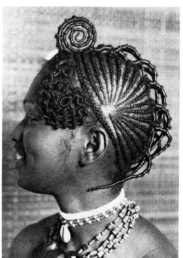

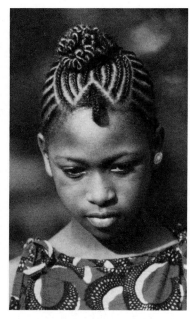

134 *opposite top right*
This style is made up of twenty-six rows of braids. The first row is braided from the front and along the hairline to the back. On each side the hair is braided upwards and the loose ends are threaded in the *Bubbled Sungas* design and joined together.

135 *opposite bottom right*
A complicated style combining cornrowing, multiple *Okoto* rosettes, the spiral motif and the *Bubbled Sungas* design.

136 *opposite left*
A combination of basic cornrowing, chainbraiding and three spirals threaded in the *Bubbled Sungas* design.

137 a & b *above and right*
Hair threaded in the multiple *Okoto* design is combined with cornrowing.

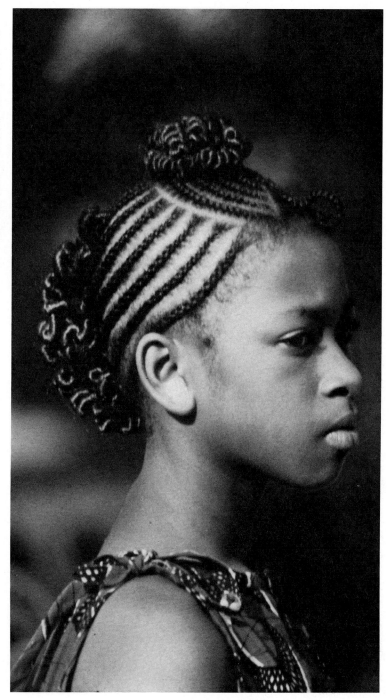

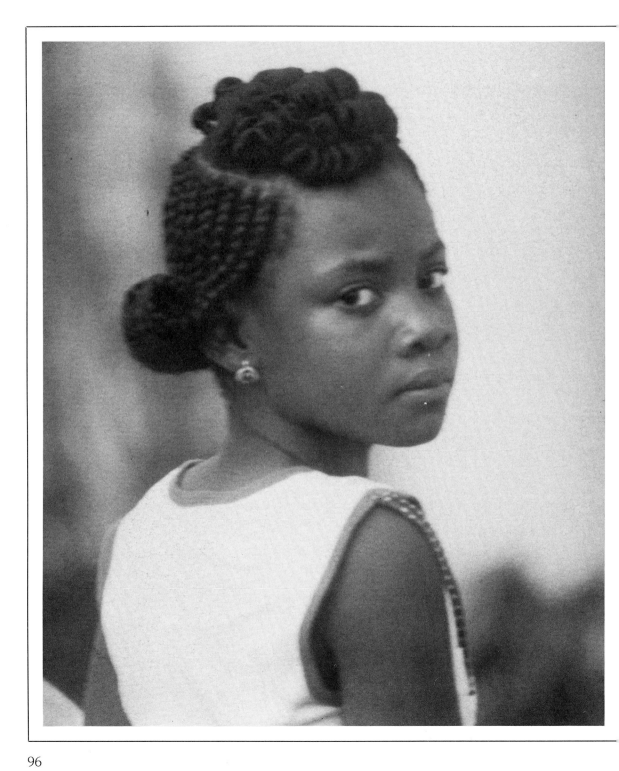

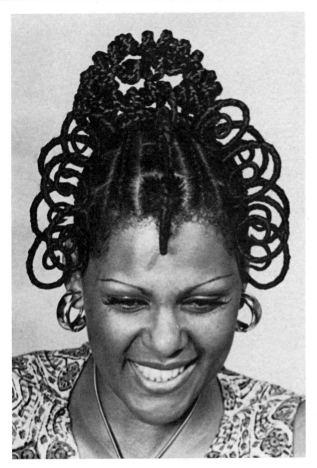

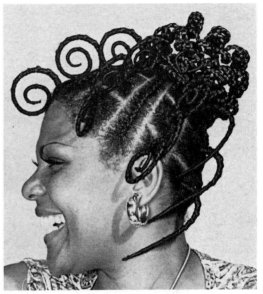

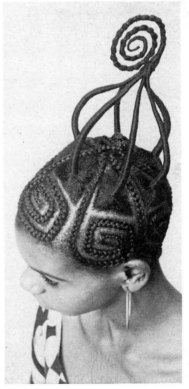

138 *opposite*
Cornrowing with an attachment is shown in detail in **79**. Here the style is combined with hair threaded in the multiple *Okoto* design.

139 *right*
Cornrowing is combined with the *Onigi* style of threading. Then at the end of the *Onigi* a spiral is threaded in the *Bubbled Sungas* design.

140 a & b *top left and right*
An arrangement combining several styles: cornrowing, threaded ringlets in the *Bubbled Sungas* design and a braided hairpiece arranged into curls.

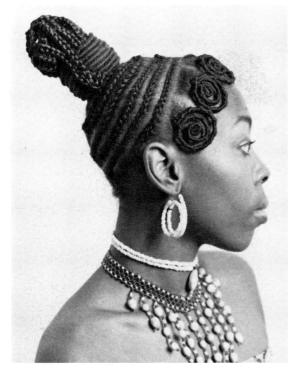

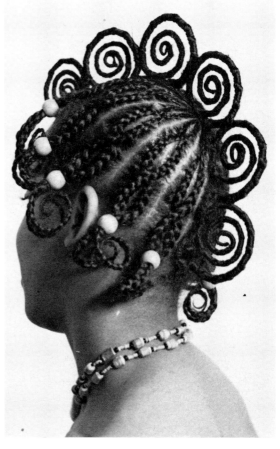

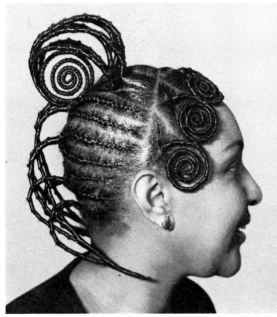

141 *top left*
The hair at the front is parted and
each section is wired, threaded and
arranged in flat ringlets. The
remaining hair is braided in circles
and a hairpiece is added to the top.

142 *bottom left*
Threading in the *Bubbled Sungas*
design combines with cornrowing to
produce this style.

143 *above*
Chainbraiding using beads for
decoration combines effectively
with the spiral design.

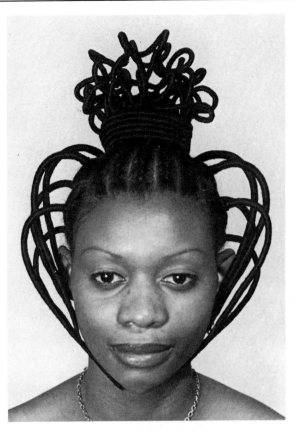

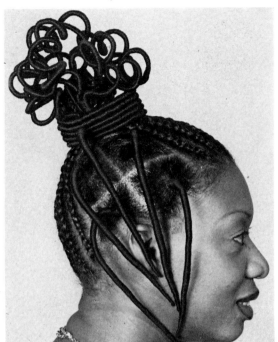

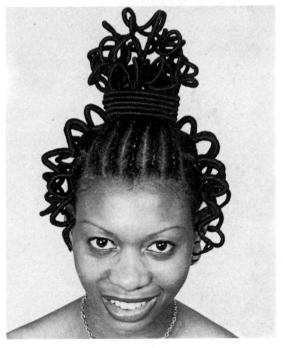

144 a & b *top left and right*
A combination of cornrowing and the basic *Sungas* design. A hairpiece threaded in the *Snake* style is added to the top of the head.

145 *right*
The same style as **144** except that the sides have been twisted into the *Snake* design with the aid of a pencil.

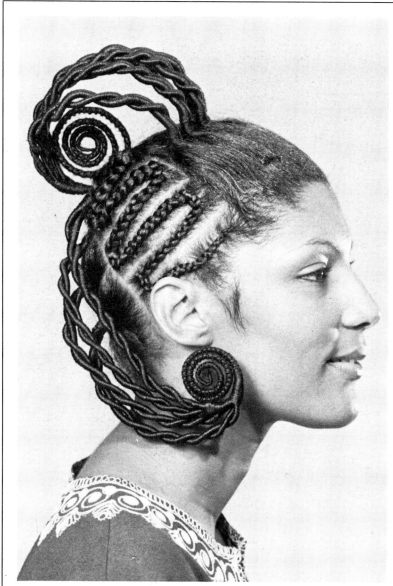

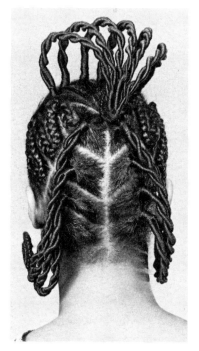

146 a & b *above and left*
The *Twist* design ending in a spiral
combines with zig-zag braids.

147 *opposite*
The *Eko Bridge* style, shown in **109**
and here combined with
cornrowing.

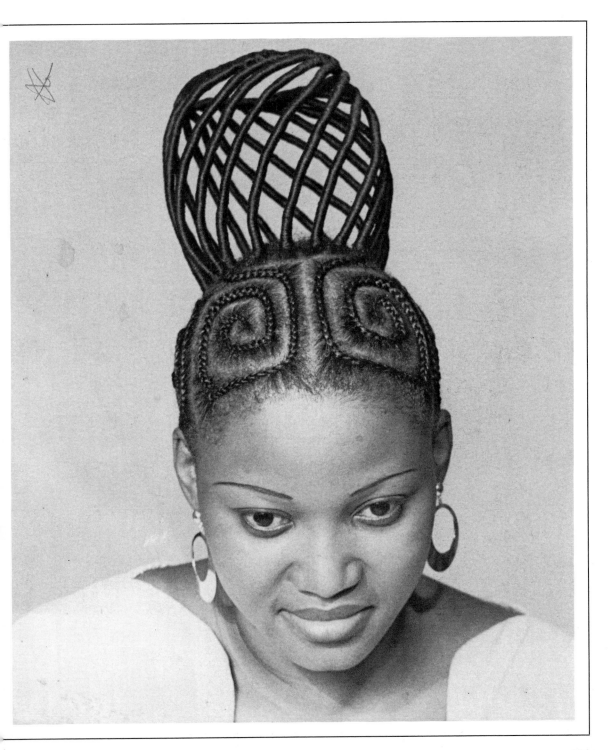

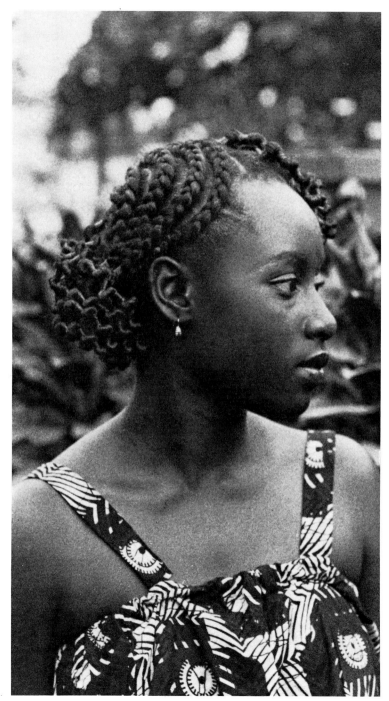

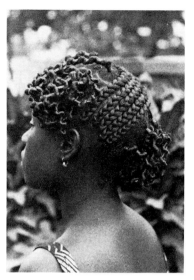

148 a & b
A style showing hair cornrowed with an attachment and hair threaded in the multiple *Okoto* design.

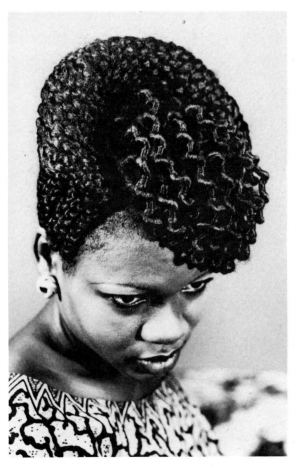

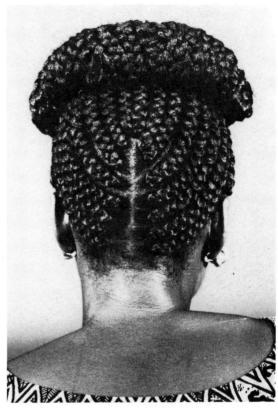

149 a & b
Another style combining
cornrowing with an attachment and
threading in the multiple *Okoto*
design.

Haircare

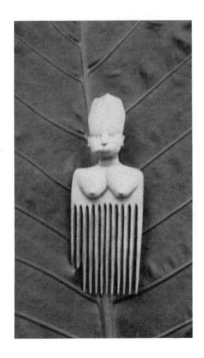

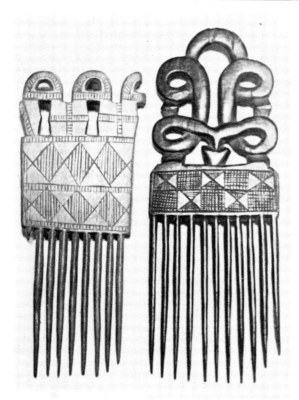

Haircare Yesterday

For men and women, an abundant and healthy growth of hair has always been most desirable. Various hair grooming recipes have been ingeniously concocted through the ages for the purpose of increasing the length, thickness and sheen, and for repairing natural defects of the hair. There is evidence of hairdressing oils and remedies for unhealthy hair dating as far back as 3500 BC in the tombs of ancient Egyptian kings.

In Africa, the main remedies used were animal fat, shea butter, coconut oil and palm kernel grease – all locally extracted from animal and plant oils. Most African women washed their hair with *ose dudu* meaning 'black soap' in Yoruba. Most old women insisted that this soap, made from a mixture of palm oil and palm husk ashes, was very good for the scalp.

150 *previous page and above*
Traditional combs.

Haircare Today

In recent times the quality of hairdressing has vastly improved owing to technological advances and the availability of newer raw materials. There is an abundance of these products available and popular brand names can be found in exclusive salons in London, New York and Paris or the remotest market stalls in rural Africa.

The three main essentials, however, for a healthy head of hair are shampooing, oiling and physical fitness.

Shampoo As the hair is constantly exposed to dust and air pollution, it should be washed as often as is necessary with any kind of non-irritating soap or shampoo. The intervals between washing should be set by how quickly the hair accumulates dirt or dandruff. As people react differently to shampoos, it is impossible to prescribe a

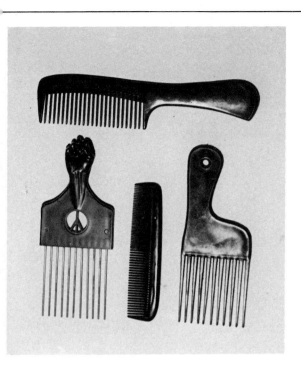

151 *above*
Modern combs.

particular brand or general recipe as being good for all types of hair. It is, therefore, best to select shampoo according to the condition of the hair.

Pomades After the hair has been washed, it should be scrupulously oiled with a suitable pomade, again depending on the condition and quality of the individual's hair and scalp. Today, there are an endless range of effective hair pomades, creams, liquids and oils on the market known for giving the hair and scalp nourishment and lustre.

Physical Fitness In addition to washing and oiling the hair, it is of vital importance to keep physically fit, eat a balanced diet and get enough sleep to ensure a healthy head of hair.

Bibliography

Arnot, D.W., 'The Far-Flung Fulani', in *Nigeria*, no. 75, December, 1962 (Lagos).

Balandier, George and Maquet, Jacques, *Dictionary of Black African Civilization* (New York: Leon Amiel, 1974).

Basden, G.T., *Niger Ibos* (London: Seeley Services & Co., 1938).

Boucher, Francis, *20,000 Years of Fashion* (New York: Abrams, 1967).

Cole, Herbert M., 'Vital Arts in Northern Kenya', in *African Arts*, Winter 1974, vol. VII, no. 2 (Los Angeles: University of California Press).

De Negri, Eve, 'Nigerian Body Adornment', in *Nigeria*, 1976 (Lagos).

Elliot, H.F.I., 'The coiffure of the Masai Warrior', in *Tanganyika Notes and Records*, 1948.

Grenfell, George, *George Grenfell and the Congo*.

Illustrated London News, 'The Mangbettu', 1929 issue.

Jefferson, Louise, *The Decorative Arts of Africa* (London: Collins, 1974).

Laugel, S/s Lt. and Marcais, P., 'Les coiffures a Tindouf', in *Revue Anthropologique*, 1953, pp. 113-21.

Leblond, Marius-Ary, 'La coiffure feminine a Madagascar' in *Le Monde moderne*, Paris 1907, pp. 533-8.

Salvadori, Cynthia and Fedders, Andrew, *The Maasai* (London: Collins, 1973).

Severn, William, *The Long and Short of It* (New York: David McKay, 1971).

Sieber, Roy, *African Textiles and Decorative Arts* (New York: Museum of Modern Art, 1972).

Smend, Von, 'Haar und Kopftrachten in Togo' in *Globus*, Braunschweig, 28 April, 1910.

Torday, Emil, *Camp and Tramp in African Wilds* (London: Seeley Services & Co., 1913).

Tyrrell, Barbara, *Tribal Peoples of Southern Africa* (Cape Town, South Africa: Gothic Printing Co., 1968).